"*Facing the Cognitive Challenges of Multiple Sclerosis* has an important place on the bookshelves of people with MS. Whether or not you are dealing with cognitive dysfunction (or are not quite sure), this is a heart-felt description of the daily struggles, the small and large losses, and the (sometimes embarrassing) emotions tied to the mental and physical challenges of MS. In the end, it is also a story of quiet victory and dignity in the face of this disease. I am very glad that I read it. You will be, too."—About.com

"Powerful and revealing, [Gingold's] is a story of denial and then acceptance, but with no hint of surrender . . . He understands that each person with MS is unique and lays out a series of steps that allows people to find an individual path. He challenges us to have four goals: get educated about the cognitive changes in MS; take action to make the necessary adjustments in our lives; reach out for available answers; and leave room for 'slow hugs."—*Inside MS*

"One of the best books [written on the subject] in some time. The writing is smooth, making his experiences visual so the reader can share in his private, cognitive struggles. Good read, especially if you suspect or know you have cognitive issues. This book helped me understand what could happen, how I could cope with it, and certainly that I was not alone in the anguish. It will help anyone with MS, their spouses, friends and physicians."—*MS World*

"The story [Gingold] tells is honest, intelligent, and often humorous. Throughout the writing he notes facts about MS and strategies for acknowledging and coping with the cognitive changes MS may impose. Readers with MS may relate to and learn from his experiences, while readers without MS may better understand the effects of cognitive issues and how one feels to suddenly encounter these perplexing symptoms."—*The MSAA Motivator*

"Language laced with ironic humor and crisp images of a mental wheelchair express the devastation of what [Gingold] terms "smack-in-the-face" cognitive symptoms . . . Gingold's memoir is . . . a poetic testament to one man's courage."—Consortium of Multiple Sclerosis Centers

"Gingold's thorough research and compassionate voice will resonate not only with fellow patients, but also with their friends, families, and physicians . . . He anticipates and answers tough questions with candor, sympathy, and a surprising amount of humor; expertly debunking the shame and frustration commonly associated with the mental ramifications of a terrifying disease . . . Insightful and informative, Gingold's guide is a much needed resource for the often invisible side of MS."—*Kirkus Reports*

"Not only does this book explore the frustration and fear that accompanies living with cognitive symptoms through a very personal lens, it also offers practical tips and perspectives on coping with a myriad of symptoms, as well as navigating such issues as decisions about medications and communicating effectively with your health care professional. *Facing the Cognitive Challenges of Multiple Sclerosis* is a book that will be of interest to anyone who would like to learn more about cognitive symptoms and the impact that they can have, but it also offers lessons in moving forward against the odds."—Multiple Sclerosis Society of Canada

"Mr. Gingold's personal account is a courageous, compelling, and revealing look at the cognitive difficulties accompanying the physical challenges of MS. It is my hope that this book will both validate for patients and their families these more subtle yet devastating symptoms, as well as mobilize physicians to more seriously consider cognitive symptoms in their diagnostic work-up and comprehensive care of their patients."—Dr. Bradley J. Fedderly, Member, Board of Directors, American Academy of Family Physicians

"Unfortunately, the cognitive effects of MS, although very real, are rarely discussed . . . Mr. Gingold's compelling and personal discussion about the cognitive effects offers new information and insights into a very real symptom of the disease. I believe *Facing the Cognitive Challenges of Multiple Sclerosis* will draw an eager and large readership seeking new information and resources."—Colleen Kalt, President and CEO of the Wisconsin Chapter of the National Multiple Sclerosis Society

"This book gives an excellent insight into how Jeffrey Gingold learned to accept the limitations of MS and found coping mechanisms to lead as "normal" a life as possible. I found it extremely illuminating with regard to "cognitive" problems that had been largely ignored for years and has put my mind at rest about the way I have learnt to try and not overstretch myself to minimize their impact."—Beryl Rice, Multiple Sclerosis Society (United Kingdom)

"The 140 pages (including a list of further useful reading) are easily read, highlighted with helpful tips, lots of examples, a great deal of, dare I say it, food for thought!"—Jenni Hall, Multiple Sclerosis Society (United Kingdom)

Facing the Cognitive Challenges of Multiple Sclerosis

Facing the Cognitive Challenges of Multiple Sclerosis

Second Edition

Jeffrey N. Gingold

demosHEALTH
New York

ISBN: 978-1-936303-20-5
E-ISBN: 9781617050879

Acquisitions Editor: Noreen Henson
Cover Design: Carlos Maldonaldo
Compositor: S4Carlisle Publishing Services
Printer: Bang Printing

Visit our website at www.demoshealth.com

Medical information provided by Demos Health, in the absence of a visit with a healthcare professional, must be considered as an educational service only. This book is not designed to replace a physician's independent judgment about the appropriateness or risks of a procedure or therapy for a given patient. Our purpose is to provide you with information that will help you make your own healthcare decisions. The information and opinions provided here are believed to be accurate and sound, based on the best judgment available to the authors, editors, and publisher, but readers who fail to consult appropriate health authorities assume the risk of any injuries. The publisher is not responsible for errors or omissions. The editors and publisher welcome any reader to report to the publisher any discrepancies or inaccuracies noticed.

The names and other identifying characteristics of some of the individuals in this book have been changed to protect their privacy.

Library of Congress Cataloging-in-Publication Data

Gingold, Jeffrey N.
  Facing the cognitive challenges of multiple sclerosis / Jeffrey N. Gingold.
    p. cm.
  Includes bibliographical references and index.
  ISBN-13: 978-1-936303-20-5 (pbk.)
  ISBN-10: 1-936303-20-5 (pbk.)
  1. Gingold, Jeffrey N.—Health. 2. Multiple sclerosis—Patients—Biography.
3. Multiple sclerosis—Patients—Mental health. I. Title.
  RC377.G56 2011
  616.8'34—dc23

                                              2011014696

Special discounts on bulk quantities of Demos Health books are available to corporations, professional associations, pharmaceutical companies, health care organizations, and other qualifying groups. For details, please contact:
Special Sales Department
Demos Medical Publishing
11 W. 42nd Street
New York, NY 10036
Phone: 800-532-8663 or 212-683-0072
Fax: 212-941-7842
E-mail: rsantana@demosmedpub.com

Made in the United States of America
11 12 13 14 15   5 4 3 2 1

Especially for Terri and her unflinching love and honest feedback, for Lauren and Meredith with their inspiring smiles and sweet hugs . . . holding close. Mickey, too.

Contents

Foreword   xi
Preface   xiii
Acknowledgments   xv
Introduction   xvii

CHAPTER ONE
"Hollar," if You Need Me   1

CHAPTER TWO
The *Knock* at the Door   13

CHAPTER THREE
Music and Mirrors   27

CHAPTER FOUR
Unanswered Questions   41

CHAPTER FIVE
It's in the *House*   51

CHAPTER SIX
The Family Mask   67

CHAPTER SEVEN
Feeling the Edges   85

CHAPTER EIGHT
Don't Just Stand There . . .   97

CHAPTER NINE
Taking the Middle Fork   117

CHAPTER TEN
Drifting and Dragging in a Mental Wheelchair   129

CHAPTER ELEVEN
Come Out, Come Out, Wherever You Are   143

CHAPTER TWELVE
In the Game   153

CHAPTER THIRTEEN
A Team Effort   165

CHAPTER FOURTEEN
Gathering New Pieces   181

In Summation . . .   195
Resources   201
Index   205

Foreword

No one who has met Jeffrey Gingold or heard him lecture can fail to be humbled by his energy, commitment, and courage in pursuit of his aim to share his experience of cognitive difficulties in MS. This book delivers that message to a much wider audience. It provides a source of information, comfort, and inspiration to people with MS who want to learn more about how MS can affect their thinking, remembering, and other abilities. It offers explanation to family members and other loved ones. It brings insights to health professionals working with people with MS.

Jeffrey Gingold's unflinchingly honest account of his journey with MS will resonate with many readers, although he stresses that everybody's experiences will be different. Cognitive difficulties are one of the hidden symptoms of MS, not always talked about or acknowledged in clinics, not always addressed or understood by those around the person with MS. This book deals with the confusing and undermining incidents that preceded the realisation that cognitive difficulties were part of his MS. Jeffrey Gingold narrates how he found expert help, which enabled him to develop and recognise his own expertise in managing cognitive difficulties and other aspects of his MS. He recounts his struggles at work, his decision to change his occupation, and the compromises and benefits that has involved. He tells of his work with other people with MS and how helpful that is to both those seeking his support and to him. Perhaps most importantly, he describes the impact on his family life and the strength he draws from his wife and daughters. After every ordeal and disappointment, comes recovery of spirit and steps forward.

There is a great deal of wisdom in this book. There are practical tips, guiding statements that frame positive attitudes, and encouragement to constructive action. Every page has precious advice for those whose lives are touched by MS. Jeffrey Gingold describes a resolute, realistic, and always positive approach to the cognitive challenges of MS. There will be many who find that this book helps them follow that path.

Dawn Langdon, MA, MPhil, PhD
Trustee, U.K. MS Trust
Reader in Neuropsychology
Royal Holloway
University of London
Egham, Surrey
United Kingdom

Preface

How would you handle getting lost while driving home—only blocks from your house? Would you be able and willing to explain it to your doctor? To your friends and family? Your spouse? When I was first diagnosed with multiple sclerosis (MS) in 1996, I envisioned being physically disabled, relegated to spending family time and a successful legal career in a permanently seated position. I never anticipated that MS would also include an invisible disability, a "mental wheelchair" that would confound my recollection and distort my rational presence of mind, turning court appearances and the routine moments of life into mental quicksand.

MS is a disease without a cure and of the 400,000 people in the United States who are currently diagnosed with MS, more than half will be blindsided by a *stealth* disability lurking within this devastating chronic disease: cognitive difficulties. This book is written for you because you or someone you care about has MS and may be experiencing this problem.

Without warning, many people with MS are suddenly faced with an inability to process routine thoughts. Their decision making may be stonewalled, befuddling simple conversations into a word-finding struggle. Others may lose their bearings in their own backyard or kitchen, or suddenly the face of a spouse or friend will appear unfamiliar. Then, the shroud over their memory recall lifts, defying explanation, and leaving no trace of the bait and switch. The individual's cognitive functions have been compromised and often go undiagnosed, creating a deep chasm of unseen disability.

As I struggled to understand my lost thoughts and stalled thinking, I looked for information, but could not find an in-depth book that offered a first-person, patient's perspective on the mental difficulties experienced by many people with MS. This book fills the void as an open memoir, candidly engaging the isolating cognitive challenges of MS. My hope is that this personal story is a clear and sharing voice that embraces all those in the MS community who are affected by cognitive challenges.

Those of us with MS who are affected by cognitive difficulties must first be able to identify and come to grips with the difficulties of memory recall, visual-spatial distortion, and thought derailment, and then accurately describe them to their doctor, before we can be treated with medication and other therapies. The anecdotal style with which I have shared my MS-related thinking difficulties will hopefully help others with MS to recognize similar changes within themselves and learn how to cope with cognitive dysfunctions. I have provided simple organizational strategies and a tactical outline for living each day fully. My slightly irreverent viewpoint is intended as an antidote for the panic and hopelessness that is often involved when fighting the mental difficulties of MS. While I may prefer not to take myself too seriously, MS deserves informed attention and action.

This book, with its pragmatic view of cognitive issues, is directed as well to the doctors, neuropsychologists, occupational therapists, and other MS-related professionals seeking to comprehend the cognitive distortion that can occur with MS. Bringing these professionals directly into the mind of the disease will foster more accurate strategies for diagnosing and coping with the mental obstructions of MS.

As a volunteer Peer Supporter for the National Multiple Sclerosis Society and presenter at the Newly Diagnosed MS Conference Series, I have spoken to hundreds of people with MS regarding their cognitive challenges, offering my personal experiences and strategies for living beyond MS. With this book, I hope to do the same for you.

Jeffrey N. Gingold

Acknowledgments

I deeply appreciate family and friends, whether offering a hand to stand up or the patience to allow me to slow down, reschedule, and adapt, encouraging me to openly share my experiences.

For Noreen Henson, Tom Hastings, Dr. Diana Schneider, Edith Barry, and Demos Medical Publishing. Also for Paul Sommer, Pamela Raglin, Amy Hempstead, Bonnie Perkins, Noelle Holly, and Biogen Idec, who have provided tremendous support for this writing, bringing MS cognitive difficulties into a public discussion. For Jonathan Siade-Cox and Jennifer Wenzler, bringing MS education directly to the people. Also for Jessica Bryan who helped me to focus this message, which can be shared with other MS patients, their families, and treating doctors.

To my literary mentor, Kurt Chandler, who encouraged me to develop my writing with simple honesty and to stop writing like a lawyer.

For all medical professionals like Drs. Matthais and Thomas, because of their comprehensive understanding of both the cognitive and physical aspects of MS, where the means of treating a patient's disability and quality of life is as varied as the individual. For all therapists who help knock pieces back in place or find the best way to loosely tape them together.

And for U.S. Speedskating Olympians: David Cruikshank, who has shown me how to move forward and give back, and Jilleanne Rookard who has taught me to not second-guess myself. For Marv Hughes and all the good days.

I am grateful to the Wisconsin Chapter of the National MS Society, especially its President Colleen Kalt, along with Mary Hartwig and Beckie Thompson, for providing the spirit and push for everyone involved in the effort to educate, support research, and find a cure for MS. For Diane Baughn, for encouraging me to share my path as a volunteer Peer Supporter. To Renee Vandlik, opening the door for me and many others to advocate for those who truly deserve a better way to exist, removing barricades, building alliances, and taking it to the streets.

Introduction

[In] most of the patients affected by multilocular sclerosis who I have had occasion to observe...there is a marked enfeeblement of the memory; conceptions are formed slowly, and the intellectual and emotional faculties are blunted in their totality.

Jean-Martin Charcot (1877)

When does the wheelchair get delivered? How many years do I have before taking a more permanent seat? When I was diagnosed with multiple sclerosis (MS), I began to ask myself these types of questions. Whether walking through a mall as a shopper, or as an attorney striding through familiar courthouse halls, I could sense the presence of a walker or wheelchair. *Was it coming for me?* I wondered. The literature about MS was clear—the majority of those diagnosed would require some form of mobility assistance within 10 years of diagnosis, and most of the rest within 25. After 5 years of quietly living with the knowledge that I had MS, my balance, vision, and mental and physical fatigue were all problematic, but I was still standing.

Although I believed that my denial about MS was under control, I was blindsided by a subtle, yet powerful manifestation of this crippling disease. It hit without warning one day in court, hiding itself under the guise of MS-related fatigue.

I was presenting a client's motion for contempt against her former partner that related to financial matters. During the prior 2 years, I had become very familiar with the history of Ms. Bartley's case, because she frequently and often spontaneously dropped by my office to discuss her ongoing financial difficulties. The hearing would be routine, because I regularly appeared before Judge Dreyfus and understood the open rhythm of his proceedings.

"Mr. Gingold," the Judge asked from the bench, "from your perspective, what do we need to do here today?"

Without warning, I was suddenly unable to answer. My prepared opening statement was gone from my mind. I was blank, void of all thought. The written phrases on my yellow legal pad were completely foreign. I turned to glance at my client in an effort to jar my opening lines, but her face was also unfamiliar. She tilted her head to look at me, waiting for me to speak. But I could only stare back, stunned by my *loss of presence* and unable to grasp my purpose. The growing silence in the courtroom underscored the problem as my desperate mind grasped for any notion of what was going on.

I was trapped! But where?

Even my trial-reflexes were unable to grasp my purpose at that moment. My brain was completely overloaded, blocked, and unable to process the prepared facts, issues, rationale, analysis, and conclusion for my client's hearing. It was clearly my move, and when the silent stares turned into murmuring, I understood that I needed to dramatically and immediately do something. Adjusting my tie, I took a deep breath and turned toward Ms. Bartley.

"You've been living this," I said to her in a subdued voice. "Just tell the judge in your own words what you have been going through. Keep it short and don't get too hot about it," I cautioned. (The court's transcript merely reflected a discussion off the record between me and my client.) Having taken the opportunity to rip open his mail, the Judge had been patiently waiting for my response.

"I'm going to ask Ms. Bartley to speak," I said to the court. As she spoke, I continued to scan my notes, pulling on phrases to slip back into the present context. Her story was familiar, but I couldn't get in front of it or keep up with the facts of her case. It was as if I was hearing it for the first time, except it did not stick in my mind. *What was I supposed to say when she was finished talking?*

My notes were waiting for me. Recognizing my own handwriting, I discovered questions that I had prepared in advance for the other party. The phrases made sense.... *I'm back!* Mentally returning in time for cross-examinations and closing arguments, the hearing was concluded with the Judge granting our requested contempt orders and other relief sought by Ms. Bartley, but I knew this was no way to practice law. My client and I had been lucky, this time. The only difference between us was that she didn't know it.

Normally, I would be pleased with my lawyer-self as I walked through the front door of my firm. Skipping the telephone messages waiting for me at the front desk, I marched straight into my office and closed the door. I continued to hold the doorknob, pressing the door closed as if something was following me and trying to slip in behind me. Slowly turning around, I faced the case files stacked on my couch. They were just as I had left them before the hearing.

Despite my mental lapse, the hearing and my reputation had been saved by a clever courtroom maneuver. As I sat down behind my desk and began to examine my calendar, I wondered what would trigger this type of bewilderment again. *What might I be doing the next time my brain tumbled into empty space?* Fortunately, my career didn't involve landing commercial airliners.

Losing myself in the middle of a hearing was not the limb-numbing symptom of MS I had anticipated. It was, however, only the first of many smack-in-the-face cognitive symptoms that would slice into my work and family life. Unlike other individuals who are disabled by the devastating effects of MS, the physical obstacles alone would not end my legal career and disrupt my life.

Facing the Cognitive Challenges
of Multiple Sclerosis

CHAPTER ONE

"Hollar," if You Need Me

The salesclerk was asking me to leave! Just spin my wheelchair around and get out of the store without touching anything, banished like a biblical leper. I had been deceived by the newly laid cement ramp that provided easier access from the parking lot to the front entrance of the mall. Now, it seemed more like a means to quickly scoot us out of the way of the "normal" shoppers.

Our group of young adults in wheelchairs was on a shopping mall excursion. We evoked a wide range of reactions and glares from each passerby, as well as a low level of fear from various store personnel, who seemed to be wondering what to "do about us." This had been especially true in 1976, a time well before the issues of disability access had been made into law. The Vietnam War and Watergate were over but not yet understood or accepted as history. Busing urban schoolchildren was the new effort to ensure that the freedoms of the civil rights laws of the '60s were a little better than the paper on which they were printed. Some of those same buses were now specially fitted for another freedom, the right to travel for those limited by their physical disabilities and environmental barricades. For me, shopping in this manner was an experiment.

Although it was only early June, you could already feel that high humidity was in the summer forecast. Then there was the "wheelchair stick factor." When seated, your clothes would absorb the moisture in the air and trap it between the skin and blue vinyl fabric of the seat. If you were able to stand, the resulting soaked clothes would look as though you had walked backward in the rain. Add one more factor: the wheelchair-rigged, yellow school bus transporting us to the shopping mall was not air-conditioned, and because it had started to drizzle outside, the windows remained shut. We were locked down in a terrarium on wheels.

With the exception of the first few rows, which were used to seat camp staff, all of the seats had been removed to maximize space for wheelchairs. The staff examined their clipboards and chatted about the timing of drop-offs and pickups, subconsciously twisting and tilting their bodies with the direction of their conversation. Our two rows were strapped in facing each other with chair wheels locked and affixed to the bus. It didn't seem fair that in a rollover bus accident we would hang safely attached upside down, while the staff would be flung through shattered windows because their seats had no belts.

Because our Easter Seals summer camp group numbered more than 20 wheelchairs, we were split up into three buses and were headed to three different malls, perhaps for ease in bus ramp access. We presumed that this was not an effort to spread our paltry cash more evenly throughout the city, but rather to avoid overwhelming one shopping mall like waves of invading Sherman tanks. Despite the large size of the school bus, it could only safely accommodate 8 wheelchairs.

After the bus pulled up to the main set of doors for the Southgate Mall, the driver opened the large exit door in the middle of the bus and pulled forward a 10-foot metal ramp from the hidden slot built under the floor of the bus. Judging by the clenching of his face, the weight of the ramp must have become heavier as he pulled to the rhythmic clicking sounds of the drop metal steps. Our wheelchair locks were released one at a time, and we were pulled through the side exit and rolled down the ramp. The driver was careful to rest each foot on a center step, while also lining up our wheels on either side of the step holes. Drivers are rarely assigned to the same bus route, and the seated individual in a wheelchair must have blind trust in the nameless stranger's grip strength, coordination, and training.

We were soon assembled on the cement landing near the mall's front doors, allowing shoppers to deliver disconcerted glances at the sound of clashing metal foot rests. We remained assembled far left of the three sets of entrance doors, while the other civilians seemed to drift far right, as if searching for the doors located farthest away from us.

A light rain hastened the staff's eagerness to gather our belongings and safely escort us into the mall.

"Be back at this entrance in two hours sharp or get back to camp on your own," Bob said, with all the authority of an Assistant Camp Director. His empty threat was delivered with a reassuring smile. Bob was a slightly curved 5 feet 7 inches and in his mid-30s. He had ignored the heat, and wore long, dark blue pants with a multicolored paisley shirt. Slightly rumpled, the collar was uneven, like his gait.

Although it was still morning, Bob already looked drained by the humidity, and it took some effort for him to stand and walk. Limping allowed him to keep a natural pace with our wheelchairs. One of his legs seemed to turn out, so that his feet were not parallel, causing the turned foot to drag a bit when he walked. Bob's unique position in understanding the challenges of people with disabilities made his counseling especially respected and reassuring.

One of the staffers held the mall door open, and I felt my wheels bang over the threshold. When the rubber on my wheels caught the well-worn carpet of the mall, my enthusiasm for shopping began to wane. The traction was thick, and it was like trying to roll through half-dried tar. Gliding from a push was not possible. Every yard of wheel turn was a hard press. A sudden fast press and the wheels would slip with no grip of the ground. I proceeded slowly and with caution.

My first stop was the watch counter of a jewelry store. Although I could not peer down into the display case, I assumed it was the watch counter because of the revolving watchband case perched on the top. One of the two male employees was changing a watch battery at an elevated table, while the other showed earrings to a young lady. The two men wore identical dark brown pants, off-white, short-sleeve, dress shirts with neck-tight, earth-tone ties, and they had bright red faces. A sign apologized for the heat, warning that the store's air-conditioning was broken. I struggled to spin my wheels against the short-shagged carpet. They both watched my slow-rolling chair without shifting their heads. Our eyes did not meet.

I could feel the warmth of the store's intense floodlights on my damp hair and shoulders. Heat rose from the glass case as I placed my hands on the metal edging and leaned forward to lift myself slightly from the wheelchair. I would just need to get up 10 to 12 inches for a good view of the pocket watches. I had cash in my pocket and felt like a customer.

The challenges of disability are not always understood by others.

> Disability can cause frustration and anger with daily life. Have patience with yourself.

"Don't do that!" said the earring expert. "Get down!" He remained behind the counter and spoke across the store in my direction, pointing his finger at the ground next to me as if I was a dog being scolded to get off a couch. As he came toward me, still holding a pair of earrings, I looked at his face for some understanding and accommodation. Instead, he was staring down through the glass at his watches. I don't know whether he was looking for damage or missing items, but he continued to scan the contents of the case. He seemed mad, yet scared of me. Maybe both.

"I just needed the edge for a second," I said, easing back into my chair. "I'm looking for a pocket watch, and just needed to lean forward a little to see inside." He stared at my lap.

"Well, you can look or ask to see a watch, but you can't use the case to stand," he snapped. I wondered which concerned him the most: the structural integrity of the case or my fingerprints on the glass. We were at an impasse, because I could not ask to see a watch that I could not identify, and if I can't see the merchandise, then they won't see my money. The sign was correct; the store was uncomfortably hot and I decided not to press the point. There were other stores in the mall, so I left the jewelry store.

As I continued toward my second purchase goal, I noticed that the bottom of each store window was level with my lower chest. The glass of the windows reflected my rolling figure as I passed by the displays of spring-colored tennis shoes, purses, and skirts, but I was only interested in buying a new pair of pre-faded jeans. The Wooden Nickel offered the best selection.

I wheeled into the Nickel, and was confronted by rows of spinning towers that suspended hanging jean shirts and skirts. I could see shelves of folded pants toward the back of the store over the top of the displays. My size was 32 in. × 32 in.—a seated tall and thin was still tall and thin. On my third try, I finally penetrated the wall of Western plaid shirts, being careful not to catch the shirts cuffs on my spokes.

The cashier, a high-school girl with shoulder-length, dark-brown hair, wearing a tight pair of Wooden Nickel jeans, managed the register with only one hand, because she needed the other hand to repeatedly scoop her dangling hair behind her ears. She had been watching me struggle, and seemed relieved when I stopped spinning the clothes racks in an effort to clear a path. Her eyes popped when my wheel maneuver around the sock buckets caught the belt rack and sent it rocking, but I was able to grab a handful of belts, avoiding a catastrophic crash. No help here—her customer assistance ability seemed to be limited to observation.

I reached the wall of folded pants and found a pair of jeans and off-white corduroys to try on for size. The wooden, saloon-style changing-room doors were open and inviting. I stared at the bottom of the door, which only came down as far as my seated waist. I contemplated how to try on pants while also protecting my modesty. At this point, the cashier approached me as another clerk replaced her at the register.

"Can I help you with something?" she said, speaking loudly and slowly. *She must have a hearing impairment or learning disability.* I hesitated, trying to politely catch her eyes before I answered. Her gaze shifted back and forth from my wheels to my resting feet.

Just then, the other cashier held up a greenish pair of folded pants and shouted, "Price check on women's jeans!"

"$19.99 plus tax," my assistant responded. From this, I concluded that her hearing was not impaired. Her head angled at me as if she anticipated I would speak incoherently. Staring at the footrest and armrest of my chair, she continued her conversation with the wheelchair.

"I would like to try on these pants," I announced in my most normal manner of speech.

"You want to try these on?" she said, challenging my simple request by speaking even louder.

Before entering the mall, Bob had admonished us to always be respectful, because our conduct would reflect on other people with disabilities. I looked into her face and saw that she was staring unabashedly at my legs. Her gaze moved down to my feet, which were sitting on the footrests of the wheelchair. I couldn't move my head down far enough to catch her eyes.

"I only want to buy one pair and need to see which fits better. Often, the same marked size doesn't mean they fit the same." Her mouth opened slightly. She seemed to be looking around for some idea about what to say next. Then she closed her mouth, and began to look concerned, as if she was disgusted by the thought of my legs trying on the pants, which I might not buy, and then she would be forced to touch them with her hands during re-shelving. Was it my resting legs or the wheelchair that injected panic into her face?

"Bob-controlled" thoughts fumed inside me as I contemplated informing her that the wheels were not infectious and I was not a deaf idiot. "Even when sitting, I still need to wear pants," I said calmly.

She looked back at me after glancing at the changing rooms, and then cracked a slight smile of relief. "You're not gonna get that chair into the changing room, anyway." She was again looking at my wheelchair. "I don't think you should buy anything here. Maybe try another store." She was serious, and reached forward, offering to take the pants from my lap. I wanted to stand up and whip them in the direction of her face, hoping the rivets would sting. But, again guided by Bob's restrictive words, I looked at her planted legs and held out the pants.

Disability can cause frustration with daily life.

Nothing had prepared me for this type of rejection. I came to the mall to shop for a watch and jeans, not to fight for the rights of people who are disabled. My eyes felt drawn into their sockets. My stare burned into the wood-planked floor. I spun the chair around and retraced my path out of the store. I was done with this mall. I needed to regain my composure before rejoining the others at the bus. Trembling with rage, I sat motionless next to the entrance of the Wooden Nickel, contemplating the cemented prejudice against people with disabilities.

As I sat there, two silver-haired ladies approached. "I thought the blouse would be on sale," said one lady to the other. They were carrying shopping bags, and quickly glanced to the ground and fell silent when they saw me. Then they picked up their casual pace and began to cut a wide swath around me. Avoiding my eyes, they looked up sideways at my chair, my legs, and my face. Finished with this review, they quickly looked back at the ground in front of them, as if trying not to get caught staring.

When I finally began to relax, I pushed toward the pickup location. It was still raining, and the four staffers assisted the bus driver by holding the doors, lowering the ramp, and quickly driving our weight up the slippery ramp and back into our locked, strapped positions. My hands instinctively grabbed the wheels when I felt the traction fail and I slipped inches back.

"Gotcha!" the driver rumbled in my ear as he retreated to a lower step. Another push and I was thrust through the open hatch and parked against the only remaining wall belts. I was the last camper on board, and I rolled into a disheartened silence that muffled the air like the steam shrouding the windows. The gleam of raindrops rested on the hair and faces of everyone in the bus as it roared out of the parking lot.

Although two or three of the campers had returned with shopping bags hanging over their handlebars, the rest of us were item-less. The tone of the conversation rose quickly to disgust and anger over the similar treatment that most of us had endured. As the bus jostled and accelerated down 27th Street, I released the safety belt of my chair.

I stood up.

None of us who were in wheelchairs were actually physically disabled, nor had we ever before encountered the world from a seated-only position. We were all counselors-in-training, and this was a clandestine educational opportunity designed to give us unique insight into the needs and expectations of our campers. Our eyes were wide with frustration. As I walked toward the staffers sitting in the front rows, two others who had also released themselves from their chairs followed me.

"Now, let's go back without the wheelchairs and see their faces," I said, turning to see heads nodding and defiant smiles. "I need to talk to some salesclerks about people with disabilities," I said to Bob, loud enough for everyone on board to hear.

Someone yelled, "Let's go!"

Bob had anticipated our reaction, and his calm demeanor met our tension. "What about the next person in a wheelchair who goes into one of those stores after you've mopped the floor with a clerk?" he said. "I doubt they'll be magically bestowed with respect and courtesy because of your comments. If we let the Southgate employees know about our training exercises, they may treat shoppers who do have disabilities even worse. This training is for you, not them!"

"Just because you think that you don't have to take their crap," Bob continued, "doesn't mean that the person after you will be able to deal with it. Think about that." His eyebrows lifted with understanding, and the firmness of his voice suggested that he had been here before. Not wanting my sweaty shirt to be stuck again to the wheelchair, I remained standing for the duration of the ride back to the camp parking lot.

The education was obvious to us, the new summer counselors at the Hollar Park Easter Seals Camp. The narrow-minded people at the Southgate Mall would require much more education than we could offer. We had already mastered transferring wheelchair-bound adults and children into the pool, bus, toilets, showers, and rowboats. But, what I also learned that day was that I had no tolerance for those who naively stare and talk down to people with disabilities merely because of their appearance.

My "seated" perspective and attitudes were chiseled into me during that hot summer of 1976, along with the insensitive faces of the salesclerks. However, I had a narrow view of how disabilities can dramatically alter a person's life. Having a disability is never one-dimensional.

As a result of this "educational opportunity," I resolved that I would never be in a wheelchair as a result of a disability—never. I actually believed I could control my destiny. The campers at Hollar Park had disabilities for life, but I had not been born that way. I had experienced both worlds, but I lived in the world without disability or a wheelchair.

From that time on, I took every opportunity to correct anything I perceived as being "unfair" to people with disabilities. It was a naive reaction fueled by my experiences that sweltering summer as a camp counselor, and later as an attorney with a progressively disabling disease.

With this indelible awareness, it became uncomfortable to be a silent witness to the micro-injustices inflicted on people who are disabled. However, working with people with disabilities and being sensitive to their challenges would neither protect nor prepare me for my own future disability.

By 1988, I had three university degrees, but nothing had changed. I was chained to working long hours as an attorney. I watched the same clock as the law students who studied around me at the Marquette University Law Library. I was in my suit all day, and had been an attorney for almost 2 years, but my hours remained unchanged from when I was a law student.

My mentor at the law firm was immersed in litigation and tactically relentless. Sensing my desire to have a life outside of the practice, he took me to the lounge across the street from our office for a drink.

"You can't walk away from the case by going home for dinner," he lectured. "It must be that important and totally consuming. If you want to take on the litigation teams of the big firms, then you must be obsessed by the case until you go to bed at night." His voice rose as he spoke passionately about the level of intensity necessary to win. "You need to be so preoccupied by the fear of what you might miss that you need that glass of wine at the end of the day if you want to sleep."

I nodded to show understanding, but not acceptance. I was mortified by the concept of "Work until you must drink." What toll would this take on my sanity and body? There certainly are better techniques to practice as a successful attorney, but once in the "Golden Handcuffs" of a legal career, most lawyers stop looking for them unless compelled by outside forces. Unknown to me at the time, I was carrying a career time bomb.

It was false advertising. *Perry Mason* only dealt with one client at a time, and only when the charges were dismissed would he move on to the next ready and waiting case. There was no law school class to warn you that half of your time would be spent on efforts to sustain your career, including networking with professionals and clients, balancing case and law firm management, court preparation, and state bar activities.

Mr. Mason's legal career was myopic and far removed from the truth. In law, it is vital to process information and make yourself clear to others. It's difficult to see an attorney's work product. They do no construction with their hands, nor do they hire the workers, but they represent those who do. Lawyers need to mentally absorb all of the details of every case and become a factual expert. Many attorneys find themselves representing 50 to 100 clients at one time. Each case is a world unto itself, with separate court hearings, intense objectives, tangled facts, witness preparation and anticipation, understanding the demeanor of the judge, and filing written briefs, cross-briefs, motions, and numerous exhibits. The raw essence of litigation is paying attention to multistressed detail, further straining a neurological crack.

By the summer of 1995, I had reached the apex of multitasking. My litigation practice seemed self-propelled, and my free time was consumed by volunteer opportunities with the state bar, board positions with local arts groups, and our first daughter, Lauren, who was now 2 years old.

"St. Mary's Hill" was located near our home, and it was so steep that snow fences were erected in winter to break up the sledding run. In summer, bolting up the hill with legs and feet turned out provided the necessary painful resistance, mirroring the starting seconds of my speedskating time trials. When the oval speedskating ice at the Pettit Olympic Training Center was melted down at the end of the season, my cross-training moved to the seemingly vertical "Hill."

A runner ran past me at the top of the hill as I neared it for the fifth time on a steamy, 85-degree July afternoon. "There are stairs over there," he offered, nodding his head toward the cement steps located 15 feet to my right.

"Thanks," I grunted back. I continued to look down for traction, knowing that he had missed the point of my workout. My legs became unusually rubbery as I tried to gracefully run down the hill in order to then begin my final ascent. *It must be the heat*, I said to myself.

Litigation meant stress, and athletics burned it away. But my perspective was shortsighted and miscalculated. I would not be able to prepare myself to run through or around the MS minefield because I carried it within me, making it unavoidable.

◆ ◆ ◆

Forced by MS to retire after only 13 years of practicing law, I was becoming very comfortable wearing Levi's jeans, Docksiders, and no socks. My goal had once been to obtain enough suits so that I could be in court for 2 weeks straight without repeating an outfit. Clothing bearing Armani, YSL, and Geoffrey Beene labels filled the upper row of my closet. Whether it was for a judge, juror, or client, I used to think it was important to look fresh, professional, and successful. I had never worn my *Sergeant Pepper's Lonely Hearts Club Band* tie to the office or courthouse.

Years later, I would realize that these suits are too nice to be left hanging in the closet.

Now, when I opened the closet door in the morning to grab a light gray, speedskating sweatshirt, I would look up at the row of suits. Hanging still and quiet for months, the suits were probably also wondering, *How did this happen?* Most people, including our children, were unaware that I had MS and had retired from my law firm. After all, I was only 41 years old and I "looked just fine." They did not understand that the mind can also be affected by MS and that these symptoms can be just as disabling as the physical challenges.

"It seems really odd to wear these clothes again," I said to my wife, Terri. "I feel like I'm dressing formal for the first time, although I have worn this suit a 100 times."

"You look very nice," she said. I wasn't sure if she was reassuring me because I was going to a funeral, or if she fondly remembered that I used to look like this 6 days a week. I reached for the front-door knob and quickly let it go. Confused, I spun around and saw my two little girls putting on their coats. *I guess I don't need my briefcase this morning.*

"You almost forgot to take someone with you to work," said Meredith. On her way to the door, she had placed her Beanie Baby kitten in my hand. Living in her 5-year-old's world, she was unaware that it had been months since I had suited up for clients or for a court appearance. Now, wearing a suit punctuated the end of my career.

When MS forced me to hang up the lawyer suits, it was an unanticipated, crushing blow. Looking back, I know that although walking away from my career was not anticipated, it was the right decision. I had no regrets about stepping off the "career rug," rather than waiting for it to be yanked out from under me. However, in order to give up my litigation career, it was crucial first to acknowledge that MS was affecting my family life and career—in time to do something about it. Family is everything and it was absolutely worth protecting my ability to be a vital part of it, by learning to deal with my MS.

> The early symptoms of MS may be subtle, confusing, and have unpredictable timing. It may take a while for you or your doctor to recognize it as MS.

The decision to retire took considered time and the welcomed involvement of some trusted individuals to help guide me through some uncharted MS territory. It would be a shocking break from life plans and without warning or explanation; it would batter me to my knees and leave me to question the very core of my sanity.

Tips for Living

- ◆ Anyone who becomes disabled probably has preconceived ideas about what life with a disability entails. It may be best to let go of these ideas and move forward.
- ◆ Evaluate early on what is most important in your life, focus on it, and let go of the rest.

CHAPTER TWO

The *Knock* at the Door

I felt as if a 30-pound child was wrapped below each knee. The light of early dusk shimmered off the mist drifting in from the wide riverbed. I wanted to escape my dragging legs and meander with the cool mist. Many people probably have had nightmares like this—they need to run after something, but their legs will only move as if they were wading through sludge.

We had only covered 200 yards when my energy suddenly ran dry. "Sorry," I said to my wife, Terri. "We need to turn back." I was feeling increasingly weak, and the inability to control my body was more than disappointing, it was perplexing.

We were on a 16-day vacation in France and, after escaping the oppressive heat of Paris, we were staying at a bed-and-breakfast in the bucolic Loire Valley. It was the summer of 1995, and there were no clients pounding on the door or children needing attention. Instead, we encountered a single powerful knock that cracked our complacency.

The early symptoms of MS may be subtle and confusing.

Back on the edge of the bed, I was relieved to be sitting. Our evening stroll had resulted in overwhelming fatigue, diminished sensation, and lack of coordination. My mind raced, searching for the cause of the shutdown. I had not been in an accident or suffered any injuries; I had no pain of any kind; and I had no answer for the concerned expression on Terri's face.

"Can I get you anything?" she said.

"You can do one thing. Kill some of the overhead lights; it's hard to keep my eyes open because of the glare."

"I think you're ready for bed," she said, after turning off the lights. I was not sleepy, but I felt exhausted. As Terri read her book under the nightstand lamp, I lay motionless next to her on the bed staring at shadows on the ceiling. We had traveled to Blois, France, because of its central location in the Loire Valley. For more than a year, we had studied photos of the sprawling Cinderella castles sprinkled around the Loire River. We had anticipated exploring three castles the next day, from turrets and dungeons to moats.

"It must be the Paris heat catching up with me," I said softly, "nothing more. Nothing wrong with crashing; it's a vacation." The tone of my answer did not project a great deal of confidence. Truth be told, I didn't know why I felt so strange. Rolling away from the open window to shade my eyes from the reading light, I could hear the water lapping against the riverbank.

"Maybe we should find something else to do tomorrow," said Terri, without shifting her gaze from the paperback.

Reflected by the river, the rising sun filled the room. We were both awake and looking out of the window. As a city boy, I had never slept with a screenless, open window before. But here, I couldn't imagine it otherwise. Absent the evening mist, the valley was alive with impressionist colors. Even the common border shrubs had a Monet-painted suppleness. The disturbing events of the previous evening seemed far away.

I had never felt the sensation of blood moving through my legs before, but now, as I tried to stand up, I could feel all 10 of my toes reaching out to grip the bare floor. The room seemed to move, and the instability of my balance caused me to lean my back against the wall.

"You still look a little off," said Terri.

"Breakfast is the answer." Then, remembering this was a bed-and-breakfast, I slipped into my shorts and T-shirt.

"*Bonjour, Madame et Monsieur*," said our hostess, Sophie, with much espresso in her voice. We had walked into the pages of a French countryside cookbook. Two large tables of settings lay crowded with scratch scones, individual coffee cakes, and fresh sliced fruits. Standing ready at the iron stove, Jacques pulled down skillets hanging from ceiling hooks and set them between sliced wedges of butter and a yellow bowl filled with eggs.

"*Café* or *juisse*?" said Sophie. I was relieved that she spoke breakfast English and I wouldn't have to struggle with a pantomime of scrambled eggs. Watching us over his shoulder, Jacques smiled and remained silent. The aroma of freshly brewed coffee and food filled the kitchen.

But then the room started to spin, and sitting down did not stop it from moving around me. I grabbed the table leg pressing against my thigh with one hand and held on to the edge of the table with the other in an attempt to remain upright in the chair.

The smell of breakfast began to cause a wave of nausea, comparable to crossing the high seas in a small boat. "I seem to have a crippling hangover without the benefit of the matching Parisian night. It's simply not fair," I said.

"You seem a little better, more alert," Terri responded, in an attempt to be cheerful.

Just then, Sophie plopped fuffy scrambled eggs down on my plate, followed by slices of fresh peasant bread. I felt like "French toast." The four containers of assorted fruit preserves seemed to move toward me of their own volition. I looked up and saw Sophie smiling down at the freshly landed food. She held a coffee carafe and was poised to refill my cup, but it was still full. Glancing at my place setting, she began to frown, perhaps searching for whatever had stopped me from touching my utensils.

"You not eating?" she said. Jacques tossed Terri's omelet in the air and caught it in a blackened pan. Sophie was still staring at me, waiting for an explanation. "You should eat; you so thin."

"I can't eat," I whispered to Terri. "You do it for me, before she notices." Terri quickly scooped my eggs onto her plate, while I broke apart a piece of bread to give it a used appearance and sipped bubbles from my orange juice glass. We excused ourselves under the assumed profile of hurried American tourists and fled.

An hour later, we encountered Chambord castle. I paused at the entrance to steady myself on a bench, then again on the third flight of stairs. Eventually, we had managed to explore the castle, the courtyard, and the grounds. The stunning castles of Chenonceau and Cheverny were also explored—the events of the previous *Twilight Zone* evening and the rolling sea breakfast forgotten. They had disappeared into the swift current of the Loire River.

Sometimes even doctors have difficulty in recognizing early symptoms of MS. Be specific when stating your symptoms and don't hide what you are experiencing.

"Please hold the gauze in place and sit up, slowly," said the nurse.

A few days after returning from France, it was time to give the annual pint of blood for the American Red Cross. I rolled my sleeve down over the taped white gauze and picked up my suitcoat, but when I tried to stand up, my body suddenly dragged, and my thoughts were slowed by the sudden heaviness of the room. I had never before had an adverse reaction to giving blood and refused to believe there was a problem, other than arriving straight from work and donating blood on an empty stomach—something that's ill-advised.

Several days later, I called the telephone nurse who told me: "You drank plenty of juice and had something to eat after donating. It's unusual to have a reaction that lasts for several days. You probably should see your primary physician. Maybe you have a virus."

When I consulted Dr. Miller, my primary physician, he said, "You are experiencing a type of vertigo that was probably brought on by a viral infection." I was relieved that he agreed with the nurse. "Take it easy, and this should work itself out within a few days. It's nothing to worry about," he said.

Sometimes, even doctors have difficulty recognizing MS.

We had no air-conditioning in our Milwaukee home, and the summer months simmered. Without a crack in the heat wave, the only reason to use window fans at night was to blend the stifling house air with the sweltering city air. Falling asleep was a brief departure from the heat, frequently interrupted by turning the pillow in search of the elusive cool spot.

It was often necessary to reschedule appointments and hearings because I was too fatigued to work and needed to go home and rest. I was unable to eat because of vertigo sensations, the loss of a pint of blood, and the oppressive heat had destroyed my appetite. My whole system had been weakened by illness, and although the doctor's explanation made *some* sense, it didn't make *any* sense that there was nothing that could be done. I spent the bulk of my days lying down waiting for the mystery virus to pass.

My work days were cut short. Rising off the bed to go to the office only seemed to magnify my draining struggle to balance and walk. A dent remains in the wall leading down the kitchen stairs, pressed there by my skull during a slip down the stairs. I was not mentally tired, so what was wrong with me?

Weekends were useful because it meant time off from work and there were no expectations for me to do anything. One Sunday morning, Terri and I decided to try walking to nearby Lake Park. For support, I leaned on the stroller that held our daughter, Lauren. After slumping over the handles for a few blocks, walking became an extreme strain. Letting go of the stroller, I dropped down onto a wood-slat park bench near the children's play area.

"We should go back," said Terri, "if you're not up for this yet." It was difficult to lift my head and answer. There was the recent memory of collapsing in another wooded area thousands of miles from home, but nothing had really changed.

"Leave me on the bench for a while," I said. "Just don't forget to take me home." I stared at the grass, trying to convince myself that I had control of the situation.

As the oppressive weeks of August heat turned into a crisp Wisconsin fall, my health began to slowly improve. The "virus" was easily forgotten—until one night in December. While we sat watching *The X-Files*, I complained to Terri that the 27-inch picture tube had faded out.

"The colors seem fine, but the picture doesn't seem as sharp. Kind of fuzzy, isn't it?"

The conversation continued in the kitchen, where I turned on the small color television in the corner so we would not miss a moment of Mulder's search for the truth. I paused while still looking at the small screen, and then quickly switched my hand to cover my left eye, then back again.

"Turn the lights on for a second," I asked Terri, as I continued to cover my right eye.

"Is something wrong with this TV, too?" she said, thinking that maybe I was also trying to find a problem with the kitchen television.

"No, seriously, there is something wrong with my eye. I never noticed before, but when I close my right eye and just use the left, the view is clouded over." I adjusted the lights in the room and continued to alternate looking with each eye. For a minute, I just rubbed them both, hoping the blockage was something that could be swept away, but both television screens seemed fogged by the same vision problem.

Difficulties with vision are a common symptom in MS.

The next day, I was examined by Scott Moretti, an ophthalmologist.

My vision slowly drifted uncontrollably out of focus as the dilating drops took effect, and soon I was in a darkened room for testing. The functions of my left cornea and retina appeared normal, but the cloud that hovered in front of my left eye remained unexplained.

"It's like driving on a slushy winter day and your windshield wiper fluid is empty. The wipers leave a smear of snow dirt across the windshield. You can still pick out large, well-lit objects and have some depth vision, but don't try to read the signs or make out detail. That's what my left eye sees all the time, sometimes worse."

"The problem may not have anything to do with the vital parts of your eye," said Dr. Moretti. "Those areas seem to be intact, but I can think of two other possibilities." He explained that if a mass, such as a tumor, was pressing on the back of the eye from inside my head, it could obstruct my vision. I imagined glancing in a mirror and seeing a shaved head with a "U"-shaped surgery scar. *This conversation is not real*, I told myself. A tumor—in my head?

Dr. Moretti adjusted his white lab coat and sat down next to me on his stool. "Another possibility is that it may be optic-neuritis, which can be an early indication of MS—multiple sclerosis." With that, I knew for sure that he could not be talking about me. MS did not belong in my world. I was a dad, an attorney, a speedskater on Olympic ice—these things I knew. What is a "sclerosis," and how could I have caught one, much less "multiple" ones? I had never even touched cigarettes or drugs.

"I just came here for some eyedrops or, at the worst, temporary eyeglasses." I thought about the client meeting due to occur in less than an hour. I needed to prepare the client to testify tomorrow, but everything was still a bright blur, and my eyes were bloodshot from the drops.

"I know we're in the middle of the holidays, but I would like to schedule you for an MRI as soon as possible," said Dr. Moretti.

"Since you live on the Eastside, Columbia Hospital may be the most convenient. Let's see if we can get you in before the New Year's break." His calm, matter-of-fact way of speaking allowed me to think of the MRI as if it were just another court appearance. I tried to pretend that Dr. Moretti was a client, and I was doing this for him.

"In the end, Moretti will probably just give me some eye exercises," I told Terri later when she called my office to hear the news.

"Do you want me to come with you to the MRI?"

"I don't think it's necessary. The test is at 6:00 A.M. and they won't let you sit with me during it anyway. I'll probably be done in an hour."

Being an attorney did not ease my discomfort when I signed the hospital forms at 5:30 the next morning, acknowledging and waiving claims related to a list of catastrophic disasters that might result from the MRI. *No, I don't have metal plates or pins in my body.*

The pale-flowered hospital gown was soft and comfortable, but I was not. There was a mirror in the changing room, but I turned my back toward it. Terri and I were leaving for an extended holiday weekend, and I didn't want to take this particular self-image with me. A quiet New Year's Eve dinner and the pristine beauty of new-fallen snow were waiting for us at the end of a 3-hour drive to Fish Creek, our favorite bed-and-breakfast getaway spot.

Up to this point, no one had explained to me what the letters "MRI" meant, including the technician who guided me into a dimly lit diagnostic room. While probably still in her early 40s, her tired eyes and slightly graying hair added 5 years. She looked like it had been a long year for her, too.

> Anger and denial are normal reactions to receiving an MS diagnosis. Obtain reliable information about MS, and then share your concerns with an MS medical professional and a close trusted person. Form a personal team to fight back.

"Do you know what they are looking for?" she said softly. "My doctor just wants to check out a little vision fog."

She used her body weight to shove the thick chamber door open. The smallness of the room was probably a result of the protective insulation in the walls and door. The girth of the MRI machine seemed to touch the walls, filling the room like the bulk of an ancient Egyptian sarcophagus.

"Lie down here on your back with your head toward the opening," she said. "You will hear a lot of noise in there." She held out a pair of earplugs. "These will help."

I stuffed the thick plugs deep into my ears and lay down on the padded, sliding cradle. Contoured pillows braced my legs and cushions were squeezed in around my head, pinning it against sudden movement. There could be no slight shift of my skull or the images would be worthless and need to be redone. No sniffle, yawn, cough, or sneeze was allowed. Not a twitch.

"Where are the tanning lamps?" I said, attempting a joke. I looked up into the narrow chamber tube. She smiled and slid a cage over my head.

"Try not to move," she reminded me.

"How can I?" I answered. "If I sneeze, my head will be pinched off."

My body lurched forward with the movement of the cradle pulling me into the cavern of the MRI machine. With the head-cage in place, I wondered whether this procedure could have been designed any more dramatically. There was nothing to look at, so I closed my eyes and thought about our last scuba-diving trip to Cozumel. Recalling the press of my face mask at 100 feet under the sea relieved any claustrophobic thoughts about the massive equipment surrounding my head and upper body.

Magnetic resonance imaging (MRI) is often used to view MS-related lesions in the brain.

◆ ◆ ◆

The machine came to life with a loud ticking that sounded like a multi-warhead preparing to detonate. The volume of the rapid-firing magnets was as deafening as a Who concert, and the earplugs only slightly dampened the pounding sensation. After about 20 minutes, the vault fell silent, and the sealed outer door popped open. I could hear the muffled sound of her walking into the room. Why didn't she wear a name tag? She knew my name and could see into my skull, but she had not told me her name. "I need to pull you out slightly for the contrast injection," she said. "Can you roll up a sleeve?"

"What injection?" Despite the banging ruckus in the tube, I had actually started to doze off and was uncertain as to whether I had heard her correctly.

"We take two sets of images. The second set is done after a contrast agent is injected into your veins. That will allow the doctor to see certain highlighted areas, which the first set may not have picked up."

By first pinning down and caging my body, she was wise to have not told me about this until now—because I hate needles. Within seconds after pulling the empty syringe out of my arm, the sharp taste of iodine covered my tongue, filling my mouth and nostrils. It tasted like old rust. "Am I supposed to *taste* the injection?" I said.

"A lot of patients say they taste iodine. It happens sometimes; but it should go away soon. Back in we go." She turned to dispose of the needle and retrieve tape to attach the gauze pressed to my arm. *Did she say "We?"*

The table began to jerk slightly in the chamber for different angle views. Another 20 minutes and "we" were finished. After adjusting to the sudden head-spin from sitting up too quickly, I exited the room.

She was sitting at a control panel staring at a computer screen that displayed my fresh images. "Can I see the pictures?" I said.

"No," she said, and stood up to block the monitor. "We are not allowed to show patients the images and can't comment on them. Your doctor will be mailed the results sometime next week. He can also call on Tuesday and have the results read to him over the phone."

And Happy New Year to you, too, I thought.

"My follow-up appointment is Wednesday, so, he'll probably call," I told the nameless technician.

It seemed cruel to conduct medical testing and then leave the results lying in a drawer for a few days. Dr. Moretti had given me the choice of a wheelchair or brain surgery as possible options to ponder over the New Year's holiday.

Would our lives be the same when the snow began to melt in the spring?

The following Wednesday, January 3, 1996, I was back at Dr. Moretti's office.

He left the room to call for my MRI results and then came back holding handwritten notes. "The MRI picked up some small lesions in a couple areas of your brain," he said. "They are consistent with MS."

I took a deep breath and stared at the floor. The news surprised and overwhelmed me. The report couldn't be accurate! I took the tissue he held out to touch my welled-up eyes. He began to explain the neurological symptoms and course of MS, but I had difficulty concentrating on his words. "What am I supposed to do next," I said, still looking at the floor.

"At this point, I think we should bring in a neurologist for a more detailed review of the MRI," he said. "Multiple sclerosis is different for everyone, and it doesn't mean an immediate end to anything," he said calmly. I thought about being immobilized and death. *What is MS?*

"However," he added, "it's not a bad idea to begin looking at your priorities and what you plan on doing years from now." This was too much honesty. I imagined being in a wheelchair at Hollar Park, except now I was the camper and there would be no standing at the end of the day. *Is multiple sclerosis a disintegrating disease similar to ALS, or a quick strike like a paralyzing accident? Am I going to die?*

"My priorities? We're expecting our second child in June." Our eyes met as I took a deep breath. Future images of tossing a softball in the backyard with our children flashed through my mind. I saw myself running alongside of Lauren, steadying her as she learned to ride her bike.

"A neurologist will look closely at your MRI, and give you some answers about where this may be going." His comforting hand remained on my shoulder as I left the exam room and returned to his patient-filled lobby.

Stunned, I walked outside into the burning glare of a cloudy day wearing sunglasses to protect my eyes. Sleet began to pelt my face as I squinted to find the car door lock with my key. Once inside the car, I sat motionless with the engine off.

"No!" I screamed, slamming my forearm against the side window. I refused to accept it. Fortunately, the sleeves of my winter coat protected the glass and my arm. My bloodshot eyes could be concealed from the office staff by hiding in my office, but returning from "running an errand" with a bloody arm would have been awkward to explain.

Anger and denial are possible reactions to receiving an MS diagnosis.

The wallpaper and dark furniture in my office conference room diffused the glaring ceiling lights. After checking out the least blinding spot in the room, I asked the receptionist to bring in Mr. Mallory, and we began to discuss the strategy for his court hearing the next morning. Throughout the discussion, the legal note-pad in front of me remained blurry and empty.

"Is something wrong with your eyes?" he said, tilting his head to get a better look at me.

"As you probably already guessed, my eyes are strained from being up all night looking through your file." He laughed and pointed at his bifocal glasses, which explained his familiarity with eyedrops. The lingering effect of my visit to the eye doctor was nothing new to him.

After the meeting, I walked down the filing-cabinet-lined hallway to my office. Paulette was paging me over the office intercom.

"Terri is on line 115," she said.

"Thanks. Put her through." There was a slight click on the telephone, and I could hear the background sounds of Terri's kindergarten class. "Are you in earshot of kids?" I said.

"They are reading with my assistant. How did it go this morning with the doctor? Sorry for interrupting you, but I've been waiting to hear and didn't know when you'd be going to court."

Since slamming my arm against the car window earlier that morning, there had been no time to think about the diagnosis of MS. Thoughts of this inconceivable news had been severed from my normal workday by jumping into a meeting. It was like a leftover fragment of a bad dream, a nightmare scene in a movie we had rented, or, more likely, something tragically unfortunate that always happened to someone else.

"The good news is that it's not a brain tumor," I said. "But, they saw something on the MRI that looks like MS, whatever that is."

"MS? What is that? What are you supposed to do? Do you feel all right?"

"Other than not being able to see clearly, I feel fine. Moretti wants me to go to a neurologist who specializes in MS. He'll talk with Dr. Miller and get a referral."

My telephone buzzed, indicating there was another call waiting.

"Do you want me to leave school early?" Terri said, "Maybe I can get someone to take over my class this afternoon."

"Thanks, but there's no need. I'm still going to the ice after work, and the coach is expecting that I'll be speedskating with the pack tonight. Other than feeling ticked off and maybe a little in the dark about spelling the word *sclerosis*, I feel fine. Why go home and worry?"

"Did Dr. Moretti say anything else?" My phone buzzed again with another page.

"He said something about getting priorities in order, but not in a dying sort of way."

"Maybe we should talk more about it after dinner," Terri said.

We hung up, and a few minutes later there was a knock at the door, followed by the sound of someone calling my name. Whoever it was probably thought it was important. My right hand tightly clutched the baseball given to me by Director David Ward during the filming of *Major League*. He often carried it during "takes," perhaps to release tension. But one night toward the end of filming, he tossed it to me. For 8 years it had been my litigation hardball, always resting on my desk and patiently waiting for my tension-releasing grip.

"Jeffrey?" queried the secretary outside the door. "Are you in the middle of something? Terri is on the phone again."

I answered with the launch of a split-finger fastball against the solid-wood door. Whack! The ball ricocheted and disappeared under my desk. The door was hushed.

Then, picking up the call, I said, "I'm sorry about this. You didn't bargain for this sort of news, especially right now." I could hear her breathing into the phone, and with the sound of her breath came a silent embrace.

Denial is a reoccurring reaction in dealing with a diagnosis of MS. Share the truth about your MS with supportive friends and family.

Although it felt as though nothing had changed, I couldn't absorb the sensation that everything had shifted. Even if imperceptible to those near me, the ground upon which I stood was shaking. Anticipation of unpleasant change filled me, as if I were bracing for the impact of a vehicle while passing through a crosswalk. I couldn't, and didn't, want to think about MS.

A child's voice shrieked through the phone.

"I should let you get back to your class," I said. "And I have people waiting."

The phone was quiet.

"I love you," she said.

"I love you too."

Tips for Living

♦ As you enter the world of doctors and medical testing, remember to ask questions if you do not understand something. Ask further questions if you don't understand the answers you are given.

♦ The physical symptoms and exacerbations of multiple sclerosis may vary in their degree of severity, as well as the consequences for each patient.

CHAPTER THREE

Music and Mirrors

Within a couple months of being diagnosed with MS, I received a letter from the Wisconsin Chapter of the National Multiple Sclerosis Society (NMSS) offering a series of meetings for individuals who were newly diagnosed, like me. The group met in the upstairs lounge of a local church. The facilitator was a therapist named Chris, who had been first diagnosed with MS in the 1980s after losing her vision. Her sight had eventually improved, but she walked slowly and with noticeable effort.

People with various early forms of MS entered the room, each accompanied by a "support" companion. As introductions began, it dawned on me that the face of MS in this room was primarily female. I was the only male in the room. When it was my turn to present my background, diagnosis, and current condition, I said, "I just want to be sure about something. Are these meetings open to both genders?" Not sure about the tone of my comment, I watched as their confused smiles slowly circled the room. Terri shifted in the seat next to me.

Support is critical for people with MS.

"Yes, but about 75 percent of the people with MS are women," Chris explained. It was a sobering comment. The women looked at each other in confirmation.

"You should know," I interrupted, "that I was sent here to represent the 25 percent of the male population who could not attend because they are in denial." Some of them chuckled. I shifted a little closer to Terri on the couch, and decided to keep my mouth shut.

Over several weeks, the group reviewed topics ranging from employment rights and symptom management to medication therapies and filing for Social Security Disability. It was reassuring to know that there was an available source of support and information.

There was no immediate reason to stop running or speedskating, so I didn't. So far, I had experienced only some vision loss in my left eye and balance difficulties. The brochures mailed to me by the NMSS discussed the unpredictable course of the disease. They covered the progressive deterioration of functioning limbs and the loss of sensation and control over various body parts. There were articles and advertising for medications that could slow the onslaught of disability. There was no cure yet, but these new drug therapies offered hope. The back pages were filled with tactful ads for equipment that might be needed to adjust to dependency when the symptoms of MS became more advanced.

I didn't want to admit it, but I felt tired and unfocused once or twice a day. Pulling myself together for a court appearance and dragging back to my car afterward began to occur more frequently. It was worse on warm, humid days in situations without air-conditioning. I felt as though my entire body downshifted in reaction to any rise in temperature. Same clothes, same office, courtroom, and clients, but I would overheat and slow down.

> Symptoms of MS include both physical and mental fatigue. Your MS may not be limited to one or the other.

My weight remained the same, but my legs were heavier to lift and my toes didn't clear the ground, causing me to trip. It was difficult to hide the stumble when the file in my hand sprawled across the floor. The flying papers were like sending up a flare, drawing unwanted attention to my shuffled walk. I tried to lift my thighs a bit higher in order to keep my toes from catching the ground. It was classic MS fatigue, and denying it merely added to the problem.

"Here are some written materials and video tapes about Avonex®, Betaseron®, and Copaxone®," said Dr. Lazow, the neurologist to whom I had been referred for treatment. "Look them over and select one of the injectable medications to start." She had a sharp Eastern European accent and blunt bedside manner.

"But I don't feel so bad," I said, slowly taking the stack of offered materials off the corner of her desk. "I don't see the point of taking such drastic steps."

"Even if there are no symptoms," she continued, "some doctors recommend that medication begin immediately."

It seemed too extreme, especially to deal with random sensations of fatigue. Other than saying what "some doctors" do, she did not explain why I should begin injecting myself. When pressed for a reason to justify the benefit of starting medication, Dr. Lazow seemed to have a "take it or leave it" attitude. It didn't add up. Maybe more espresso would be similarly beneficial? There seemed to be no urgency to start taking medication, and Dr. Lazow's ambivalent tone made it easy to ignore her suggestion.

As for my difficulties at work, she told me to stagger my appointments and deadlines, and to work longer weekends. She said I might be tired, and that I should find time to relax and stay in air-conditioned rooms. It sounded simple enough, and we installed air-conditioning at home.

I had a normal attorney workload: an average of 75–100 cases. It was an endless, moving line of changing names, facts, and court deadlines. Whether it was legal analysis in preparation for an oral argument or glancing through transcripts, I couldn't keep up. My concentration waned and stalled as I opened and closed file folders, searching for a simple legal task that I could complete. Despite the need for more intense scrutinizing of documents, often involving reading to myself aloud, the forced repetition of thoughts felt as though I was trudging through thickening mud.

There could be no laying back or allowing others to perceive any slowdown. Opposing counsel and support staff, as well as clients, are sensitive to such changes in the dynamics of representation. People would know that something was wrong. Disclosure of MS and its potential impairment could start a domino effect. Cases and clients would be compromised and lost. What affected me also affected my clients, my career, and the success of my law firm, with a final impact on my family and its multifaceted existence.

Denial is a reoccurring reaction in dealing with a diagnosis of MS.

It became increasingly difficult to separate physical fatigue from what felt like mental fatigue, if such a thing was possible. My thoughts began to drag, and it was difficult to absorb even the simplest information. My mind was busy with: *focus on sitting up straight, keep eyes wide-open, lift both knees to avoid drop-foot stumbling, and show a confident smile.* It was a strained balance, perhaps similar to trying to handwrite federal legislation while scuba diving on a half-tank of air and watching for sharks.

In hindsight, it made no sense to mix MS with a litigation career. It was a recipe for a scalding boil-over. The shadow of denial was close at my heels, making me believe that I could deal with this—just take the hits and keep moving.

"Could you repeat that?" I would ask others during the course of my work. This was my new method of delaying information so that I had enough time to understand it. I was easily distracted during conversation or writing, and incoming details entered like a flood of debris, passing through and sometimes clearing out other thoughts along the way.

"Please take a message" was another technique. My assistant developed a knack for running interference for me, answering potentially high-stress calls and organizing clients' financial forms and details. She would get the information from me, and keep it moving until I was able to focus. She thought I was overbooked on court appearances and took on too many of the clients' emotional problems. I allowed the office staff to believe it was that simple, in order to avoid discussing my MS diagnosis.

◆ ◆ ◆

Rob, one of my partners, stormed into my office and slammed the solid wood door behind him. The lay of his loosely combed red hair could be used as a barometer for his intensity. When bothered, random flurries of his hair contrasted with his usually controlled, corporate attorney demeanor.

"You are the most arrogant bastard I know!" he said, his volume carrying through the door and most likely out into the rest of the office. Leaving my fingers on the computer keyboard, I turned my head to see his flared face staring unblinkingly at me in his most intimidating style.

"I didn't have time to take the call," I said, ignoring his comment and tone. "Sorry you had to grab it." My need to take *one thing at a time* was the reason, but he didn't understand my difficulties in meeting anticipated deadlines while also handling other clients.

"This response brief needs to get written and filed downtown by 4:30," I continued. It wasn't an apology and Rob wanted to kick something. Having no time or patience for a further showdown, I met his stare. "Is there anything else?" I said.

He spun around and stormed out of my office, bouncing the door off the rubber stop on the back wall. Rob didn't understand that I was overwhelmed by my normal workload, because he didn't know I had MS and couldn't break my writing concentration to take a simple phone call.

The inevitable day came when I was forced to reveal the truth. It was becoming increasingly difficult to function, and I had become withdrawn and defensive with my colleagues. My law firm partners, Rob, Doug, and Michael, entered the conference room. They seemed curious about my impromptu request to meet with them. The conversation was awkward as we assembled around the conference room table.

"Every time we gather unexpectedly like this and close the doors, the staff thinks someone is being fired," Doug said, breaking the tension.

"Thanks for coming on the spur of the moment," I replied. I stared out of the window at the snow-frosted trees lining the parking lot, trying to decide what to say. I felt as though I had gathered relatives together to hear the reading of a family member's will.

"Out of respect for our partnership and friendship, I need to explain what has been going on with me." They silently waited for my revelation.

"I guess there's no good way to say this," I said, hesitating for a moment, "but I've had a medical problem for the past year or so...." For 30 minutes, I explained my situation and answered their questions about my MS diagnosis, along with its encroaching effects on my family and career. The seriousness of what I was sharing struck me when I noticed Rob's eyes watering up. They also had young children, and they looked as if they were envisioning how they would feel if something like this happened to them.

"You're still a good attorney," said Doug. "Have you started to tell clients?"

"No. If you had to choose between two attorneys, and one has a chronic disease, which one would you pick to represent your case?" I answered. Why should a client risk their case with representation that may fail because of a medical condition? My Hollar Park experiences had taught me that people judge first and educate themselves later, if at all.

So, I told my colleagues, "This subject is not for office gossip or further conversation. I will not talk about it again. If I see a problem, I'll let you know. Don't bring it up." They silently stared at me out of concern. Back in the denial "closet," I heard its door slam behind me.

My daily work routine included closing and locking my office door, and turning off the lights. However, reducing the fluorescent glare on my fogged vision didn't lower the well-stacked piles of files on my desk. Glancing across the mountains of paper, I would catch a file name and try to orderly process the work waiting in the folder. Opening the file and directly examining its contents only jammed up my efforts. The ability to scan and instantly absorb information was instinctive and imperative to successful litigation practice, and things were not going well.

The timing and accuracy of details were becoming unreliable. Facing the rapid-fire moments in court or conferences became frightening. The reflexes of my mental muscle-memory had become unpredictable. It was as if an unseen force was hitting the clutch of a stick-shift car, disengaging the gears, and then urgently catching them, lurching and stalling out the engine.

The symptoms of MS include physical and mental fatigue.

MS is a progressive disease with different symptoms for each person. Learn about MS well beyond comparing yourself with others.

At appointment after appointment, Dr. Lazow listened to my complaints about my lack of concentration at work. She didn't seem to appreciate my predicament of trying to present a client's case when the information had been scrambled and I mentally stumbled. She listened, offered a sympathetic head-nod, and then moved on to the standard neurological testing of my vision and limbs. Compared with her other patients, I was still standing and walking into her lobby with no visible MS problems. With the suit and tie, I "looked fine." Maybe she should have known better.

With the assistance of the frigid air at the Pettit National Ice Center, rigorous speedskating continued to provide my body and mind with a powerful workout. On the ice, I was disengaged from the world of suits, conferences, and the demands of clients and colleagues. The ice was my sanctuary. There was only the whispering rhythm of the straightaway and slicing crossovers of the turns. Bolting through frigid air and down the endless stream of white ice required and sharpened my focus, freezing out the day's turmoil. Wearing the tiger-stripped blue and orange "skin" of the West Allis team, I was unrecognizable as a person with MS. But whoever heard of a person with MS also being a speedskater? It seemed impossible.

One day while skating, I felt a strong urge to call the Neurology Clinic at the University of Wisconsin-Madison's hospital. The long-distance number had appeared in an article announcing an upcoming medical study. It had been buried for weeks in my briefcase. I had finally realized that in order to continue my demanding law practice, I would have to fight MS. Although denial may be empowering during the initial stage of an incurable disease, it can also become a distraction that delays treatment.

The clinical drug trial proposed by the researchers at the University of Wisconsin-Madison's hospital involved the use of high doses of a laboratory-engineered form of vitamin D. The initial laboratory results were promising; lesions in mice, similar to those seen in MS, had been reduced in the study.[1] The doctors were now ready for human subjects. After hours of qualifying paperwork, telephone interviews, and physical screening, I was accepted.

"We require an 18-month commitment to monthly MRIs, blood and urine testing, and perhaps more, depending on test results," said Dr. Fleming. His straight, silver hair and soft demeanor befit his well-established reputation as a neurologist and medical advisor to the MS Society. "We have to closely monitor the vitamin D levels in your

---

[1]Unfortunately, at the end of the study, vitamin D was found to be ineffective in the treatment of MS.

body, because continued high numbers could potentially cause liver damage, among others things."

"Not a problem," I said, ignoring the 180-mile round trip and the words "liver damage."

"We want to be sure that the people in the study make the commitment to see it through," he continued. "You will be helping to determine whether this vitamin D substance can lead to a treatment for MS. Based on our testing with mice, it almost looks like a cure, but we can't be sure of anything until we see how it works in humans."

The hospital pharmacy provided the supplies, including an extended supply of daily oral medication and syringes for precise measuring. The self-reporting recordkeeping was closely monitored, but when Dr. Fleming informed me that there were no needles for the medication, I knew this was the study for me, regardless of the amount of paperwork.

There were needles, however. Sometimes there were two a day when I had an MRI immediately followed by blood testing. After months on the medication, my blood test indicated that a dangerously high amount of vitamin D had saturated my system. Dr. Fleming reduced the dosage amount and modified my eating habits in an effort to bring the level down. No milk, cheese, or any food products that naturally contained vitamin D. My coffee would now be black. With no margin for error, I was afraid to even look at a picture of a dairy cow.

Lying in the MRI chamber, I closed my eyes and listened to Mozart's *Eine Kleine Nacht Musik* through the earphones, while the magnets began to survey the lesions in my brain. The other identities that I carried during the day were shed—there was only space in the chamber for me and the MS.

"Everything still O.K.?" said Bret, the MRI technician. The sound of his voice startled me out of a slight doze. I turned my folded arm and flipped him a "thumbs-up." The room was silent again, except for the sound of the heating ventilation. The magnetic equipment firing around my body had paused. Bret entered the room to inject the enhancing solution into my arm prior to running the augmented brain scans.

His first and second attempts to inject my arm failed when the needle stuck, unable to penetrate deep enough into the vein. He stared at the used needle, while pressing gauze against the blood-tipped mark on my arm. The problem wasn't with the needle.

"Let's try the other arm," he said, as he cleaned off my arm and placed another Band-Aid on the second-effort mark. "Really sorry, but that vein is giving me a hard time and fighting the needle. Did they just take another blood sample?" I nodded my head—yes.

The bruising on my right arm was a sign of needle-resistant scarring hidden within the vein. Dozens of prior needles had marred the path, obstructing Bret's current efforts to pierce the vein. He frowned and scrunched his eyes, as if he could feel the needle tip piercing into his own arm. I glanced away from my arm and his contorting face.

"I could use a margarita," I said.

Bret laughed, and then sighed.

"Don't worry; this hurts me more than it hurts you," I said.

The left arm was impenetrable, too. "Let's try the right arm one more time?" I suggested. It felt as if a blunt pen was being driven into my arm; my face flushed red from the blood rushing to my head, and my legs shivered from the coolness of the room. I felt as if I was about to lose consciousness; then the familiar taste of iodine confirmed that the needle hit the vein.

In an effort to avoid passing out, I concentrated on thinking about my family until the machine fell silent. Bret held my forearm and supported my back with his other hand as I slowly sat up. "Give me a moment to shake off the blood rush to my head and I'll get out of here," I said.

"Are you O.K. to drive back to Milwaukee?" he said. "It's dark now and the roads are probably snow-covered again. It was a blizzard before we started."

"If you're suggesting that I sleep here tonight on the MRI tray, no thanks!"

The legs of my pants were quickly covered by fresh-falling snow as I shuffled through the parking lot. I slumped into my car seat. Unable to shake the light-headed sensation, I slowly pulled my car out of the hospital parking lot and onto the highway.

"I may be awhile," I said to Terri, who was listening to me through the car's speaker phone.

"The girls are already asleep," she said. "Are you still in Madison?"

"I'm parked at a truck stop just outside of Madison." I was barely able to force out the words or hold my head upright. "I can't drive like this." Whether it was a reaction to the "enhancing solution" or the multiple puncturing, I couldn't think clearly enough to drive.

"Should I come and get you? Should I call someone at the hospital?"

I moaned softly, while reclining my seat and adjusting my head against the padded door. "Stay put. Let's give this some time," I mumbled. "There's more than a half-tank of gas, and I can lay here for a while with the engine and heat on. The car's covered with snow, and no one will care or notice—it's a truck stop."

"Keep your phone turned on so I can call you," she said. "Don't start driving without talking to me first."

"I'm staying here and closing my eyes," I answered.

Additional accommodations were needed in order for me to continue functioning as an attorney. I had MS-induced optic-neuritis that intensified with the slightest bright light. Bright light of any kind increased the fog patch in my vision, obscuring physical perspective and printed material. Using my "good" eye in the glare of full light created further strain, which then increased the ache in my head and made me short-tempered.

I also needed to keep my office cold in order to avoid fatigue, so I had a separate thermostat and venting controls installed in my office. My temperature panel also controlled adjacent offices, freezing the occupants year round. Since my body's preference was nothing higher than 70 degrees, it had been suggested that I hang a blanket outside my door for use by anyone who needed to enter my office. Despite all of this, I still needed to step outside during January's 15-degree days, just to cool down my core body temperature, which seemed to fire up even during the shortest telephone negotiations. After 5 or 6 minutes outside, I could feel the heat deep in my body cool, and I would begin to quiver from the frost on the outer layer.

Many people with MS are adversely affected by vision difficulties, heat, and humidity, so adjust the lights and keep cool.

The office staff still didn't know about my diagnosis, and no one suspected that their attention was being diverted. My peculiar need for cold evolved as my illness progressed, but a house of music and mirrors couldn't hide the mounting desperation of my situation.

◆ ◆ ◆

"This coffee is really weak!" I said to Terri, as I poured the whole pot down the sink. "It tastes flat." I made a second pot with two extra scoops of French Roast, but it tasted no different than the first.

"Ooooh," said Terri, after taking a sip of the new coffee. "Now, that'll keep me awake for a while."

After one swallow from the fresh cup, I poured it, too, into the sink.

"Are you feeling all right?" Terri said. She knew that turning my back on coffee was a true indication of a serious problem.

Dinner was also rather bland that night, and the strawberry preserves on my morning toast tasted like fish paste. My whole tongue and the roof of my mouth were now numb. Food and liquid disappeared from detection after passing my lips, until the gentle sensation of traveling down my throat. The focus on swallowing made me uncomfortable. Watching in the bathroom mirror, I tried yawning exercises, stretching, and clicking my jaw with ear-popping force. My mouth was as deadened as a crossed leg that had "fallen asleep."

MS is a progressive disease with symptoms that are different for each person.

By the next morning, the edge of the shaving razor felt dull against the left side of my face. After repeatedly thumping my cheek with my forefinger, I traced the numbness across my cheekbone and back over my scalp. On the very top of my head, I could feel the touch of my fingertip again. The bizarre numbness had spread, and now affected almost half of my face and scalp, from the inside out. Next, I noticed that the sensation in my left hand was gone, along with my grip. No matter how much I stretched my fingers, cracked my knuckles, or shook my hand, it was numb—plain and simple. These strange symptoms seemed more like symptoms of stroke than MS.

Feeling desperate, I went to see Dr. Lazow, who offered me steroids. "Are they addictive? It always seems that professional athletes can't stop once they start taking them."

"This is different," she said. "Large doses of steroids sometimes stop the progression of numbness for a short time. You can take them for several days, and then the dose is slowly tapered down."

I left the pharmacy with a bag containing steroid pills, other pills to protect against damaging the lining of my stomach, and still others that would allow me to sleep at night. I thought about my grandmother's weekly pill container and realized she had the right idea.

Although I could not taste mild salsa or spaghetti sauce, the pills burned once they began traveling down my esophagus. The lit torch in my gut smoldered through the night, doubling me over with enough heartburn to power-up a small village.

At this point, I had no appetite and food was flavorless. Utensils and glasses slipped from my left hand. I had constant blurring in my left eye, overwhelming fatigue, and drifting concentration. But these MS symptoms were merely preliminary impediments. My experience of MS would be outside of the mainstream interpretation of the disease, and still wouldn't involve a wheelchair.

Although it wasn't emphasized in the publications, and Dr. Lazow hadn't mentioned it, I knew that, for me, MS was both physically and *mentally* numbing.

> At least half of all MS patients are affected by cognitive problems, many of them left undiagnosed. Half!!

Tips for Living

♦ Educate yourself with information from the NMSS about the symptoms of MS and their emotional impact and effect on employment.

♦ The cognitive difficulties resulting from multiple sclerosis are different from the physical problems, although the two elements can certainly negatively affect each other at different times.

♦ Learning how your body reacts to the environment and various stress factors is vital in minimizing the number and severity of MS exacerbations.

♦ There are useful things that you can do in your office, home, and automobile that will moderate the flow of information and enable you to better absorb incoming details.

♦ Make your environment as comfortable as possible to decrease mental and physical fatigue. For example, whenever possible, adjust the room temperature to avoid becoming overheated. Remember that it is often easier to slightly warm up the core temperature of your body than to rapidly cool it down after you have already become fatigued. Layered clothing can be used to adjust for changing temperature and activity.

♦ During the heat of summer, cooling vests and wristbands are especially useful to minimize sinking into mental slowness and a physical meltdown—seek shade and air-conditioning.

♦ When optic-neuritis is a concern, avoid working under fluorescent lighting and use a softening, nonreflective computer screen filter. To further ease eyestrain, adjust the fonts and the contrast of background shading on your computer until they are comfortable.

♦ Wear UV-sunglasses whenever the glare of light decreases your clarity of vision, even if it is a cloudy or foggy day.

♦ Written communications are easier to refer to later, rather than multiple, fast-talking voice-mail comments and numbers. If you are working, have your assistant take written telephone messages for you.

♦ E-mail is useful, as long as you are not inundated with spam and large numbers of messages. Limit access to your e-mail address to only people whose communications you value.

♦ Close the door. Whether for a rejuvenating nap or to limit distractions, quiet your space to increase your focus on the task at hand. Use light background sounds, such as instrumental music, to cover interruptions from extraneous conversations and noise.

♦ It is important to tell the people you are close to about your difficulties and why you need helpful accommodations. The NMSS has pamphlets about MS that you can share with those individuals who could benefit from a better understanding of your possible symptoms, including thinking difficulties.

CHAPTER FOUR

Unanswered Questions

Dr. Lazow didn't think I had much to worry about, and I was eager to agree with her. Externally, life seemed unchanged with the exception of the birth of our second child, Meredith. Doctor appointments were squeezed into my busy litigation day, and I took a black leather briefcase with me when I went. The contents of the briefcase were irrelevant to the appointments, but carrying the case into the corridors of Columbia Hospital made it look like I was on a business-related visit. I sometimes encountered clients, friends, or relatives at the hospital, and I used the briefcase as a prop so no one would know why I was really there.

Dr. Lazow clipped my last two sets of MRI images into the white-light display case. She silently glanced from image to image while I closely inspected the different slices of my brain. Even if I searched the scans for hours, I would miss any significant change between the images, but I needed to see them for myself. It was no different than if my car had broken down, compelling me to open the hood and look at the engine, although I would be totally unable to identify the broken part.

The unfamiliar images from inside my head were only pictures and didn't allow me to come to grips with the damage being inflicted by MS. The white lesions were scattered and slight in their appearance, compared with the overall size of my brain, but there was little solace in viewing their size, because they shouldn't be there at all.

"Is it possible to tell from the MRI images whether I'll become disabled?" I asked Dr. Lazow.

She glanced silently at the images of my second MRI and then delivered her conclusions with a deadpan demeanor: "Your kind of

MS is the type that shows little progression. It will plateau with few exacerbations and no real disability. It will not become much different than it is now."

I heard the words "no real disability," which, to me, meant no wheelchair, no walker, and no cane. Maybe the years of obsessive running, physical training, and speedskating had paid off. Dr. Lazow seemed satisfied that the progressing numbness in my fingers and facial muscles had been halted by the massive rounds of prescribed steroids.

If my left hand couldn't move fast enough to type my legal briefs, then I would dictate them. No one would notice the difference, and my MS would remain under control and invisible. I was physically functional enough for Dr. Lazow, but she still had not offered any insight into my thinking difficulties.

"It sounds like part of your physical fatigue," she said, during an appointment. "When your body is having trouble with MS, perhaps your mind may also be tired and need a break."

She wanted to discuss drugs. "Medication might slow down progression of the disease." This made no sense to me, especially since she had already said that my disease was not progressing. It was starting to become clear to me that Dr. Lazow didn't understand my condition at all. Why endure the possible side effects of drugs when I may not need them? What would be the point? I decided that intravenous medication was for really sick people, not me. Sometimes denial means hearing only what you want to hear.

Dr. Lazow's "treatment" was limited to scheduling appointments several months apart. She continued to test my physical balance, coordination, and vision, but we never reviewed my mental clarity. My strained thinking was outside of her standard neurological tests for MS levels of impairment. In retrospect, I realize I should have demanded better answers, but I trusted my doctor.

Consult with a doctor you trust, but also get a second opinion if you are not satisfied with your care.

Dr. Lazow missed the signals that should have alerted her to my MS cognitive disability. While the general literature for MS patients lacked specific discussion regarding these types of symptoms, Dr. Lazow should have taken them more seriously. My care had been incomplete.

I continued to press her for answers: "It's impossible to focus at work and get through a day without being overwhelmed. All I can do is close the door and put my head down. Sometimes it helps, most often it doesn't."

"Mr. Gingold," said Dr. Lazow. She paused while flipping through my file, as if trying to remember my medical history, "Maybe you should think about retiring and going on Social Security."

"What!" I screamed. "Quit my job?"

"With what you're facing, it might be wise to explore your options."

My shock at the suggestion of leaving the practice of law was exceeded only by the bruise to my ego.

InsideMS, the quarterly national publication of the MS Society, was sitting on the corner of her desk. The same issue had arrived in my mail 2 days earlier. *Dr. Lazow is a neurologist, and she is supposed to know more than a monthly summary in a magazine*, I thought. But none of the magazines I'd read said anything about problems with focusing at work, remembering details, or getting mentally jammed up. I was angry, very angry, with Dr. Lazow. How had she arrived at the conclusion that I needed to retire?

"It is difficult to know what the MS is doing," said Dr. Lazow, "but we should probably get a different look at how it is affecting you. There are additional tests to measure changes."

Now I was totally confused. None of her conclusions made sense. Appointment after appointment, Dr. Lazow had listened to my complaints, but didn't take them seriously or relate them to MS. Compared with her patients in wheelchairs, my thinking symptoms must have appeared to be minor, but they were powerful and had the potential to be just as disabling as the physical difficulties of MS. It had been so easy to accept her misinformed diagnosis.

> The decision to begin MS medication may be difficult, but it should be approached early and the available options carefully investigated with the input of an MS medical professional.

I decided to follow up on Dr. Lazow's suggestion and go to the MS Neurology Clinic at Froedtert Memorial Lutheran Hospital for neuropsychological testing.

Eleven patients sat in the Neurology Clinic's waiting room. They were solemn, glancing back and forth from each other to the floor or a magazine. Even the conversation between spouses was, at best, a whisper. This cloistered area behind a partial wall cast a serious tenor, set apart from the hospital bustle of white labcoats and gurneys.

The sound of doctors being paged over the hospital intercom mingled with the nervous clicking sounds of wheelchair brakes, walkers, and canes tapping against chair legs. As I swaggered through the waiting room, my path was blocked from the reception desk by a wheelchair sitting in the aisle. The waiting room was packed by patients' mobility-assistance devices. My suit and briefcase set me apart from the casual dress of the other patients and gave me the appearance of "working." I walked around the obstructing chair and brushed the dust mark left by its wheel off of my black pin-striped pant-leg.

"I'm here to see Dr. Matthais," I said to the receptionist. She held up one finger and answered the phone, which didn't stop ringing even while she was talking on it. Her other hand rested on a keyboard, but she nodded her head that she had heard me. Despite trying to balance so many immediate demands, her forehead and eyes remained soft. She had the compassionate face of a caregiver, and her patience was calming. "Are you a drug rep?" she asked, glancing at my briefcase.

"No," I answered, thinking that I was dressed more like an undertaker. "I have a nine o'clock meeting with the doctor."

Josie Matthais, the neuropsychologist, greeted me in the waiting room. She was younger than I expected and appeared casual and confident. She directed me to her office, where she sat down behind her desk and adjusted her shoulders, as if to match my stiff-backed attorney posture. I pulled two of her office chairs together: one for myself and one for the briefcase.

"Your situation presents a number of MS-related possibilities," said Dr. Matthais. "I would like to conduct a battery of tests to help us narrow this down. Since it's early in the day, we can probably accomplish everything today and get you out of here later this afternoon. If you get hungry, you can grab lunch in the cafeteria down the hall."

Neuropsychological testing can be used to identify the cognitive symptoms of MS.

She obviously didn't notice that I was wearing a suit, holding a pen, and taking notes on a legal pad. My calendar was booked weeks in advance. "You want me to clear my whole day?"

"If we get started soon, you may be out by four o'clock. It will save you an additional trip to the clinic if we don't have to do the testing on two separate visits," she said.

I considered the alternatives and decided it was probably best to face the potentially significant testing rather than postpone it and then wait and wonder. "Do you mean we can finish the testing today? I can make some calls and rearrange my schedule."

> Moving toward acceptance is dealing with an MS diagnosis and not surrendering to it.

In the end, the tests measured more than correct or incorrect answers. Actually, there probably were no right or wrong answers. One test, in particular, seemed to be designed to measure only one thing: whether I would get ticked off enough to walk out in the middle of the test. Some of the questions vaporized in my mind before I could find answers. The end feeling of the daylong testing was not good. The verdict from Dr. Matthais would be ready within a few days.

"Your test results are classic for MS cognitive problems," said Dr. Matthais.

"I know I have MS. What do you mean *cognitive* problems?" I had been anticipating a cane or a walker at some point in the future, but I had never heard the word "cognitive" connected to MS. "Classic" meant old cars and Coca-Cola, didn't it?

"Although your intellectual levels tested out at the high-to-superior range," she continued, "your mental processing has been slowed, as shown by the lost courtroom incident. In one particular test, it was practically a processing shutdown." The crisp clarity of Dr. Matthais's conclusion collided with my expectations, and I double-checked the door, hoping to see that she was talking to someone else who had entered the room. Perhaps sensing my opposition to her conclusion, she adjusted herself in her chair and tucked her straight dark hair behind her ears.

The phrase "cognitive problems" hung in the air between us, unspeakable and impossible to assimilate. My mental stumbling had been summarized with those two words. "The Oklahoma City bombing prosecutor has MS, and he handled the trial from a wheelchair," I said. "I doubt his brain was slowed."

About half of all MS patients are affected by cognitive problems, many of them left undiagnosed.

"That may not be his type of MS," said Dr. Matthais, "but about half of MS patients are affected by similar cognitive problems. Many physicians don't understand the connection, and their patients remain undiagnosed." My face clenched, as if facing the blunt press of a wind tunnel. "It's not easy to identify cognitive problems in MS," Dr. Matthais continued, softening her approach. "People are hesitant to mention that they are having thinking problems, especially when the difficulty comes and goes. But in your situation, it is clearly interfering with your executive functions and decision-making."

For months I had been silently wrestling with my diminished concentration and reduced work production, and now Dr. Matthais's matter-of-fact explanation revealed the truth of my nightmarish existence. She said what I had not been able to imagine or allow myself to believe. My worst fears had been brought out into the open. Unknown by me from the start, multiple sclerosis could also mean *thinking fatigue*, and it was as disabling as the physical symptoms of MS.

"We should schedule another appointment to discuss the available medication," said Dr. Matthais. "Your record shows that you're not on any of the current treatments."

"It didn't seem necessary," I said. "What's available isn't good enough. Even the manufacturers of the drugs don't seem too confident about the effectiveness of their products." Dr. Matthais tucked another strand of hair behind her ear, sat back in her chair, and took a deep breath.

"We're going to need to work on this," she said, slightly angling her head and smiling. After scheduling a follow-up appointment to discuss medical treatment, she offered to give me a copy of the thick report so that I could review it at home, in detail. I stuffed the test results and detailed diagnosis under a deposition transcript in my briefcase.

But then, after I left her office, I felt I had to read it immediately, so I sat down in an outer lobby chair and began to review it. The background discussion in the report was familiar, but the analysis and conclusion were as unfamiliar to me as correlating the space shuttle's reentry specifications to my understanding of how to fill up the gas tank in my car.

I left the hospital and headed for my car in the parking lot. It was gone! Peering up and down the aisle of cars, I felt foolish, and wearing a suit and carrying a briefcase didn't help. Scanning the parking levels above and below, nothing was familiar. The memory of parking my car and its location was completely gone from my head. Only by pacing up and down the aisles, while clicking my remote car key, did I finally trigger the familiar beeping of the vehicle. The point was well received—it's time to stop denying my situation. My life wasn't over, but it definitely was changing.

◆ ◆ ◆

"Dr. Matthais also told me to consider a different career, one without stress," I told Terri.

There, it's out in the open, but it sounds so drastic, I thought.

"Didn't Dr. Lazow suggest the same sort of thing?" said Terri.

"Yes, but she never explained why. But now, given Dr. Matthais's test results, it probably wouldn't hurt to get a copy of my firm's disability insurance policy to review. I might need it."

How could I keep working when I might blank out again in court or in the middle of mediation or negotiating on the phone? I began to contemplate the potential repercussions. I envisioned the unthinkable, perhaps similar to a surgeon who suddenly loses the use of a hand or an airline pilot who enters a cockpit unable to focus on the control panel. If I stopped practicing law now, it would be more on my terms, and not because I was reeling from a catastrophic and irreversible litigation mistake. At least it wasn't Alzheimer's disease— Dr. Matthais explained that memories and level of intelligence are not diminished by the cognitive challenges of MS.

> Taking constructive action means learning about MS and what negatively affects your mind and body.

How would I explain retirement at 41 to my staff, clients, friends, and family? Only my law partners and Terri knew I had MS. She would understand and support the decision, especially if it might slow the progression of my MS, but how do I tell our girls that Daddy is home to stay? I was standing on the precipice between the pending disaster of where I was and the unknown place I was headed toward.

After three university degrees and 12 years of practicing law, how could I just walk away from it all? It was like experiencing a train collision in slow motion, and there was nothing I could do to stop the oncoming devastation. I needed time to think it through.

Tips for Living

- ◆ First, obtain referrals to MS-trained medical professionals.
- ◆ When you consult with your neurologist, bring with you a list of questions regarding your symptoms, potential medications, and therapies, as well as a pen and pad of paper to write down the doctor's answers for later reference. Offer the doctor the opportunity to make a copy of your written questions and concerns so that they can be included in your medical records.
- ◆ If possible, bring a support person with you to your appointments to ensure that all of your questions get asked and are fully answered. Respectfully demand to be heard and thoroughly examined.
- ◆ Ask the doctor about his or her experience in treating MS patients with cognitive symptoms.
- ◆ Does the neurological examination discuss both cognitive and physical symptoms? If yes, what are the benchmarks that will be noted? If cognitive symptoms are not included in the examination, ask why.
- ◆ Ask to see your latest MRI and request an explanation of the images as compared with prior images.

- ◆ Ask about the location and size of any lesions or brain atrophy (shrinkage), and how they might relate to your cognitive and physical symptoms.
- ◆ Request an explanation of treatment options, their different benefits, and possible side effects.
- ◆ If the answers to your questions do not make sense or inadequately address your concerns, consider obtaining a second opinion, preferably from an MS-informed neurologist who is recommended by the MS Society.
- ◆ Follow the advice of your doctors and other therapists.

CHAPTER FIVE

It's in the *House*

"For starters," I said to Terri, "there are about six more appointments with Dr. Matthais."

"Will there be more testing?"

"Not yet. The doctor seemed surprised that I wasn't on any of the MS drugs, but before starting them she wants to discuss the test results and my symptoms, including the court thing. I'm sure she will pressure me into taking medication."

"You should do whatever you need to do," Terri said. "No matter what she says, the decision is still yours."

"Bringing the entire drug hassle into the house is not a cure! What's the point?"

"If drugs can help, even a little, then don't you think it's worth it? I'll help you," she offered. "I'll sit through the training and learn about the drug mixing, storage of the supplies, etc. The videos also suggested using candles, music, or anything else that makes it easier."

The decision to begin MS medication may be difficult, but it should be approached early, and the available options should be investigated carefully.

"Dr. Matthais is probably right," I said, "but she has her work cut out for her. Stubborn lawyer, you know." This was the being dragged, kicking and scratching part of *acceptance*. As inevitable as hitting the water after having leapt off a diving board, I knew where this was leading. If my days of pretending that I was a mere witness to MS must end, then I should play an active role in that decision and not wait to be told that it was too late to take action.

Reflecting back over the past year, I realized that trying harder and working longer hours provided a temporary illusion of control, but it was self-defeating. In fact, the extra effort did not make any-thing easier; rather, it accelerated my inability to respond to the most routine matters. The physical and mental symptoms of MS worked hand-in-hand as they spiraled down into an exhausting and entangled web that tightened around my mind and body. It was as if the distance between related thoughts was growing larger and larger, slowing down and disconnecting the logical sequence of my thinking.

◆ ◆ ◆

In addition to practicing law full-time, I was an Adjunct Associate Professor at Marquette University Law School. I was now on the other side of the evening lectern, unwinding after a day in court. At 10:00 P.M., the law library appeared unchanged from when I had attended school. The late night preparation for classes still required many hours of preparation for each hour of actual class time.

Teaching about the law was safely removed from my actual daily practice of law, and it was completely detached from my hospital visits and imposing discussions about MS. Printed on my Marquette staff identification card was "Professor"—not "Professor-MS."

One particular class of third-year law students met for two straight hours, one night a week. My day of courtroom and office exhaustion was stacked against their day of classes, studying, and clerking. We were halfway through an evening class, when I noticed that the room had fallen silent. They were all staring at me, but I was not speaking.

There was nothing to say to them. Not only did I not know what to say next, but I had no recollection of what I had just said. It could have been anything—an explanation about the ethical dilemmas of attorney-client retainer agreements, football playoff scores, or the expensive on-campus parking.

My class materials were neatly stacked before me on the podium, notes on the left and handouts on the right. My lecture style was simple: a few pages of notes with well-thought-out bullet points for discus-sion. But, suddenly, I could not recall what I had just said. My mind was blank, and I couldn't find any direction from the notes. The next written lecture comment was unclear, and glancing back at the material that I had just covered triggered nothing in my clogged thoughts. There was no jump-start to continue the lecture. The class waited silently for me to move on. Someone opened a soda and note pages were turning.

Having been through this mind-jam before, I knew that the mental emptiness was temporary if I could relax and let it pass, but I still had to deal with the deafening silence of the room. "Excuse me while I take off my suitcoat," I said to the class. "It's been a long day, and besides, none of you are wearing suits, so why should I?" It was an effort to stall with a confident smile, while waiting for my brain to catch up with the presentation. As I turned back to face the lecture hall of students, there was still nothing useful about the groups of words on my legal pad. Not wanting to pause again, I gambled on a "stab-in-the-dark" question for the first student who caught my eye.

"Mr. Stein," I said, "since you started law clerking, have you encountered a similar situation at your law firm?" I didn't know what the "situation" was that I had been talking about but hoped that he had been listening and would respond. As he began to speak, four other students raised their hands, wanting to add their clerking experiences to his comments. As they regaled their law firm nightmares, I flipped a page of lecture notes and quickly read through the next subject of discussion. Somehow, it all made sense again.

"Thank you all for sharing," I said, and then moved on to the next topic.

This *loss of presence* had completely erased my thoughts of the lecture. Then, moments later, the lapse in recognition itself vanished. Multiple sclerosis was advancing simultaneously from two separate flanks, but now I had a neuropsychologist who understood how to contend with the mind-bending part of the struggle.

"How often have you been experiencing these slowed recognition episodes?" said Dr. Matthais.

"Sometimes, it comes and goes once or twice a day. Other times, I get lost for larger chunks of time. Those are the disturbing and really awkward moments—suddenly losing track of what I was doing or should be saying."

"How do you survive the moment? If you don't know how to deal with these disruptions in thinking, it can slowly begin to limit your activities."

"Frankly, it has become easier to turn away from in-depth dialogues and cancel social plans, rather than physically and mentally hold myself up for layered conversations with friends," I said.

> You are not alone in dealing with MS cognitive challenges. These difficulties are commonly reported by people with MS.

It was as if Dr. Matthais had anticipated and understood my desire to avoid these experiences by curtailing activities, rescheduling plans, and shirking personal contacts. What began as a mental safeguard had quickly become a compulsion to avoid conversation. Exposing my mental difficulties was incredibly frightening.

Moving toward acceptance is part of dealing with MS diagnosis.

Although my mirror-rehearsed nods and silent smiles suggested my participation, often an exchange of words bounced off me as I studied the faces of friends and coworkers. Just recently, I had become overwhelmed at an office party.

"Is everything O.K.?" said Terri. We were at my law firm's annual holiday dinner, and I was ready to leave after only 30 minutes. "You've been hiding at this corner table since we arrived."

"I can't keep up with the conversations." Terri looked confused by my answer. She sat down next to me at the empty table. My hands were shaking uncontrollably from MS, as if an earthquake was rolling down my arms. Sitting on my hands at this suit-and-tie evening may have looked childlike, but it was the best way to quash the shuddering without shaking the table.

"Are you cold?" she said. "Everyone else is freezing and you took off your suitcoat."

I felt like my body was shaking apart and my mind was unnerved. "It's easier for me if I just sit and smile when they stop by the table one at a time," I said.

"We should go," said Terri. "You don't look up for this."

"But how could I leave?" Although listening and trying to follow the evening's discussions was torturous, I was a partner with the firm and everyone expected me to be there. It would be awkward to walk out before dinner had arrived. The white-noise of numerous

conversations numbed my thoughts to everything except noticing the slight crack in my water glass. "Let's cut out as soon as dinner is over."

"Let me know if you want me to drive." she said.

"That's not a bad idea. Just get me into the quiet of the car, and I'll be fine."

"It sounds as though Terri has picked up on your inability to think clearly," said Dr. Matthais.

"She has definitely seen it happen, although I haven't explained it to her in detail."

"Doesn't it seem like she is also experiencing your MS?" said Dr. Matthais. "Even if you never discuss it with her, she is living it through you. What would you lose if you were completely open with her?"

I was unable to immediately answer this question.

After talking it through, the conclusion was perhaps obvious, but not before Dr. Matthais had helped me to see it for myself. Terri and I were already going through my MS moments together, whether or not I knew it at the time.

Fortunately for me, Dr. Matthais did not feel restrained by the one hour allotted for each of my appointments. She approached my MS as a personal campaign. Dealing with a litigator's argumentative stubbornness would take patience, and Dr. Matthais did not waste time. She focused on answering my questions, intent on getting me to think in terms of actually dealing with the disease.

At the next appointment, she held the last series of my MRI images and offered me another copy of my extensive neuropsychological testing results. I adjusted my blue, diamond-patterned tie and held my pen to a pad of paper, as if prepared to take notes in a deposition.

"Dr. Lazow looked at the same MRI scans," I said, "and she said nothing about the progression of my MS, or that I was developing cognitive problems."

Dr. Matthais held the images up toward the light.

"I can see the lesions scattered throughout my brain," I said, "but they still mean nothing to me. Based on where the white spots are located, can you tell what their placement has to do with what has been happening to me?"

"While the correlation between a detected lesion and a specific exacerbation is not perfect," answered Dr. Matthais, "we can certainly see where the disease is active. Sometimes it's an indication of what may happen if there is new activity, or it may simply reflect what a patient is already experiencing. In your case, it may be both." She grabbed a pen off her desk and pointed at a couple of the white lesions on the scan. The medical terms identifying the affected regions of my brain were beyond my comprehension. Dr. Matthais continued to point at each spot and talk about how its location might explain either my thinking or physical difficulties.

One fact was not lost on me—there was a clear explanation for my mental stumbling. It was multiple sclerosis—maybe not the way that I had previously understood the disease, but it definitely was multiple sclerosis. For the first time since my initial diagnosis, MS became an informed, constructive discussion, but where it would lead was still uncertain.

Understanding the causes of MS-related symptoms can enable a person to take constructive action.

◆ ◆ ◆

"I don't know whether or not you're aware of it," said Terri, "but you are being very short with the kids." She paused to lean in and make eye contact. "You asked me to mention things like this. I don't know about work, but at home you've been overreacting for reasons that don't make sense. Lauren is only 7 years old. She doesn't understand why you get so upset." Terri saw what was happening, perhaps better than I did, and was correct to point it out. I became furious with any interruption or delay that might invite another lost thought.

It didn't matter that I had shunned clients' phone calls all afternoon, only to struggle with reviewing an 18-page settlement proposal. I would read a few sentences and then read it again. I brought the case file home for further review. It would be another late night.

As soon as my briefcase hit the floor in the front hallway, Meredith wrapped her arms around my legs as high as she could reach. She didn't know that fatigue had already tripped me once earlier in the day, sprawling me to grab the end of a conference room table. I desperately needed a wall to lean against, but to 4-year-old Meredith's eyes I looked like I needed a sweet hug.

From the living room, I could hear my daughter Lauren's frustration with the piano as she repeated the same line and mistake over and over.

Terri was in the kitchen answering the phone. "Do you want to talk to Tim?" she said.

"Daddy," said Lauren, "can you help me with this music?"

My coat was still on, but I couldn't remember what Terri had just said.

"Play that later!" I yelled at Lauren. "There's too *much* going on!" It was like a bad scene from It's a Wonderful Life, *and I was George Bailey but didn't know it.*

The night before, I had broken a plate by tossing it on the kitchen table. No one knew how unproductive my work days were or how concerned I was about missing crucial legal technicalities. How could they understand my difficulties? I felt like I was walking through a minefield in the dark.

"One at a time!" I insisted. "Can't we just be quiet and skip the questions?"

Both children stopped speaking and stared at me. Terri came to the door, looking concerned. "Let's go upstairs and change into jammies," she said to the girls.

I wanted to go back outside and come in all over again. No one in the house expected or deserved my frustration. Each of them had to deal with their own day without also having to handle mine.

"You're right," I said to Terri. "I get really frustrated when more than one thing happens at the same time, even if it doesn't involve me. Everything is so distracting."

"You don't want the kids to be afraid of talking around you, do you?" said Terri. This image hit me hard, replacing the children's embraces at the door, which I had been taking for granted. My confused thinking was like thickening woods closing in behind me. If I didn't deal with it soon, I would no longer be able to protect the most important thing in my life: my family.

"It's not fair to them," Terri continued. "Maybe you can talk to Dr. Matthais about it."

"You were right to bring it up," I said. "It will probably fill the next appointment. You know my old law school books collecting dust on the shelves? When necessary, feel free to throw one at me. At least, I'll get some use out of them." Terri smiled, and then shook her head at the shelves of potential ammunition filling the 8-foot-tall bookcases covering one wall.

"Should I start with the paperbacks?" she said, reaching for my forearm without losing eye contact. "Why don't you take off your coat and eat something? I was just about to go upstairs and get the girls washed up for bed."

"I'll read to Lauren tonight," I said. "It will be a good opportunity to apologize for snipping at her."

"She probably will have forgotten about the whole thing by then," said Terri.

But I won't, I thought.

Our children didn't even know what MS was, nor that I had "it." But it was creeping into their lives through me. So far, I had managed to leave my work-related tension at the office. Work stayed at work, while home was for family time. When I was home, I was home. The line was very clearly defined, and I guarded the distinction. But now it seemed that the boundary was becoming blurred.

I understood everything Dr. Matthais had said, but it was hard to accept her perspective on MS. It was like being told that I had been making payments to the wrong credit card company and now a long-ignored and overdue balance needed to be paid.

"Anger is a normal reaction," said Dr. Matthais, "especially when you can't predict or control what is happening to you. If you have a good understanding about it, you can talk about it. That is probably the biggest step in dealing with disorientation. It's easier to deal with anger when you recognize what triggers it."

Dr. Matthais wasn't telling me that I shouldn't get angry, or that I have no right to be furious when I lose control over my thoughts, but rather, that I needed to learn how to avoid transferring my frustration to the first available target. Whether I was at work or at home, I had allowed insignificant comments and incidents to set me off. I needed to choose between becoming confrontational and avoiding conflict.

"Am I really dealing with my anger and frustration?" I asked the doctor. "Terri would probably tell you that I'm acting more and more like a shut-in in order to avoid contact with other people. She takes all of the telephone calls because I won't answer the phone. At work, the secretaries run constant telephone interference for me, although they don't know the reason why. They have developed a list of legitimate-sounding excuses as to why I can't take a call."

"Has anyone asked if there is a problem?" said Dr. Matthais.

"No, they probably think that I'm taking on too much work. It isn't that the calls aren't important, but taking a call blots out whatever I was concentrating on. I can't follow the shift to the new subject."

"Is this happening just with phone calls?" said Dr. Matthais.

"Any kind of interruption confuses me completely," I said.

"How do you manage to get through the day?" The phone rang and the doctor quickly answered it. She spoke to someone about needing another 15 minutes and hung up, turning her attention back to our discussion without missing a beat.

"I was like that," I said, pointing at her phone. "I used to be able to bounce from one conversation to another without missing a beat. Now, the messages pile up until the end of the day, when I can sit quietly and return the calls. I used to be able to type a letter, talk on the phone, and respond to my secretary's interruptions—all at the same time. Now, whether it's a knock at the door or a telephone page, it's impossible to keep my thoughts on track."

Dr. Matthais nodded her head as if she understood what I was saying. "Have you considered telling your staff about the MS and your frustration?"

"Until recently, I didn't know for sure that it was MS. But, now, it may be time to open the subject."

"Their support may surprise you, but only if you level with them."

The thought of discussing my personal life with my colleagues and staff was more frightening than any court appearance. It wasn't that my privacy was so royally precious, but rather that I couldn't handle being distracted. *I needed to do just one thing at a time* and then move on. At home, I would find a quiet, dark corner of the house and just sit, often on the floor, and stare at a random object.

It was the only way to ease my mind back from chaos. When I felt comfortable, I would listen to the message and call the person back. It was a disjointed way of living, but it quickly became a routine.

"Maybe you should explain the problems you are having in concentrating to Terri," said Dr. Matthais. "She must realize that something is not quite right, even if you haven't talked about it."

Terri's comment about not wanting the children to be afraid to talk to me was in the forefront of my mind. "No, I haven't told her everything about it. I don't want MS to take over our lives. As it is, I spend too much time anticipating the next flare-up."

"Don't you think Terri should know when you are having a problem, especially if you're leaving all of the family's social contact to her? It may help her to help you, especially if she understands you are having slow, difficult moments. If you don't say something, how can she know when MS is a problem? Certainly not by just looking at you."

How could I argue with this kind of logic? Dr. Matthais was right. My silence did not protect Terri from the MS fallout. In reality, she was even more vulnerable, simply because of the fact that she didn't know what was happening to me—her husband and the father of her two children. I needed to be more honest with myself and Terri about my stalled thinking. It might be the only way to get through the mental quicksand of MS. I needed her support, and if I wanted her to be involved, then I could no longer conceal my difficulties.

After several appointments with Dr. Matthais, it was clear that, for me, MS also meant mental symptoms. This was not just fallout from physical fatigue as proposed by Dr. Lazow.

"Originally," I said to Dr. Matthais, "I understood that when MS lesions burn through the coating of nerves they sever sensation in the connected body part."

"And the nerves control everything," she added.

"But I thought MS was only a physical problem, not something that can cause confused thinking."

Cognitive difficulties are commonly reported by MS patients.

"Actually," said Dr. Matthais, "these types of difficulties are commonly reported by MS patients. Cognitive problems show up in different ways for different people. Some patients are greatly challenged by learning new things, even simple stuff. For others, following a conversation, solving a problem, or answering a question can shut them down."

"The obvious answers don't come out," I said.

"Right," Dr. Matthais continued, "and it doesn't matter how smart the person is—MS can interfere with problem-solving, the normal process of reasoning, and the speed of memory recall. The fact that your job includes the stress of being in court has only made the experience more intense and noticeable. There are studies suggesting that stress can, in fact, make existing MS symptoms worse."

Dr. Matthais wasn't surprised when I explained to her the frozen-thought incident from my recent classroom lecture. "It was like playing a part on stage, but someone had switched the play and dialogue," I said. "I had no idea about what to say next."

"That, too, is a classic cognitive symptom of MS," said Dr. Matthais.

"So where does it all end? You said 'memory recall,' but I thought MS was not like Alzheimer's, and that I would not lose my memories."

"That's right. Your memories are not lost or erased. They are still there, but it can be more difficult to remember them when you need them."

Maybe this sounded like good news for a senior citizen, but not a 40-year-old trial attorney. "Why haven't I seen any books or articles about MS thinking difficulties?" I said. "This explanation about lesions attacking the thinking areas in my brain is a shock."

"There has been extensive research and many articles dealing with cognitive disability and MS, but unfortunately the discussion seems to be limited to medical journals."

Dr. Matthais provided answers that validated my frustration, but it wasn't easy information to accept. There was also comfort in sharing incidents that I had never dared to reveal to anyone. She answered my questions with such immediate knowledge and understanding that, in comparison, the appointments with Dr. Lazow seemed like discussing my symptoms with an auto mechanic. Dr. Matthais offered answers even before I could define the questions.

Although Dr. Matthais wouldn't say anything specific about Dr. Lazow, it was clear to me that she thought Dr. Lazow had not handled my case very well. In addition to not addressing my cognitive symptoms, a review of Dr. Lazow's medical records showed that she had failed to record the steroid treatment she had prescribed to deal with the numbness in my hand, facial muscles, and skull, and my lack of taste sensations. The records did not record any of my ongoing complaints of mental difficulties and inability to think clearly. Dr. Lazow's incomplete notes were a further indication of her inadequate understanding and poor medical treatment.

I concluded that returning to Dr. Lazow for further treatment was counterproductive and pointless. The only positive thing that she had done was to refer me to the clinic and Dr. Matthais. The neurological clinic at Froedtert Hospital was clearly on the cutting edge of both the diagnosis and treatment of multiple sclerosis, including cognitive damage. I decided to seek further treatment at the clinic. "Is there a neurologist here who would be willing to tolerate an attorney for a patient?" I asked Dr. Matthais.

"We have an excellent group of neurologists, but I'll have to check and see who is accepting new referrals. Dr. Allan Thomas would be a good fit for your situation. I have worked with him on a number of similar cases."

Dr. Matthais's approach to my diagnosis and answering questions was informed and effective, unlike the time spent with Dr. Lazow. In addition, Dr. Matthais's analysis of the medical reports was thorough, and I was confident that she would refer me to an informed neurologist who understood that *MS is not limited to only physical exacerbations* of numbness, loss of vision, and balance difficulties.

> MS medications are tools of action and hope, doing something real about having MS.

◆ ◆ ◆

Although it was my first appointment with Dr. Thomas at Froedtert Hospital, traversing the facility was a familiar routine, and when I heard my name called to have my weight and blood sample taken, it felt like a natural extension of Dr. Matthais's treatment.

Dr. Thomas was in his early forties and appeared to be athletic. Despite wearing a white hospital labcoat, his quiet voice and smile made me feel that he would listen and understand my frustrating drive to continue speedskating and live my life. After reviewing my medical records and completing an extensive neurological exam, Dr. Thomas asked me specifically about the thinking problems that had been plaguing me.

"Medical studies have shown that cognitive functioning can be affected by multiple sclerosis," he said. He placed my neuropsychological test results down on the desk. "Unfortunately, you fall into that group." There was no hesitation in his voice suggesting that anything in my MS profile was strikingly rare. This was nothing new or unusual. The cause of my mental stalling and lost moments of presence was very obvious to Dr. Thomas, and his explanation was both caring and direct.

It was horrible news, yet he and Dr. Matthais had each spoken the most validating words that I had heard since my diagnosis. They confirmed that I wasn't falling apart merely because of the pressures of litigation and family life. They verified that there was a reason for my stumbling thoughts and resulting anger. This was a tangible new factor, an unanticipated element of multiple sclerosis. Dr. Thomas quietly waited for my reaction as I absorbed his statement.

"I see that you are not taking any of the MS medications," he said. "Dr. Matthais is a good person for you to work with regarding your cognitive challenges and the available medications. If we're going to do anything to slow this down, I think you should seriously consider one of the drug therapies. Fortunately, there is more than one to choose from."

This was the good news.

"I would like you to start one of the treatments as soon as possible." He looked into my eyes and nodded his head, as if waiting for me to acknowledge my willingness to start MS drug therapy. But was I willing to become an active patient? Had all of this diagnosis effort been a waste? At this point, medication involving needles seemed inevitable and essential.

"Whatever we need to do to stop this," I said, returning his head nod. "I'm ready."

What I had not initially grasped was that having multiple sclerosis was not about acquiring something. Rather, efforts should be focused on identifying and maintaining what was truly important. Recognizing those *assets* and re-evaluating their unique importance to my life would be a process, a shift in how I perceived everything. I could no longer fool myself by denying that I had MS. Despite pretending that the doctors and hospitals were merely appointments, this was not "business as usual."

At best, my multiple sclerosis was unpredictable and confusing, changing its appearance and method of attack without any warning: mind to body, then back again to mind. Answers neatly defining or predicting my MS were sparse. Like the chicken and the egg conundrum, I never knew for sure which MS symptom was causing another symptom to fire up. Were the tremors in my hands and weakened limbs caused by fatigue—perhaps set off by the stress that resulted from trying to follow conversations, or was it the other way around? Maybe my inability to follow a discussion was merely because I used so much extra energy to keep my body steady and upright. Although I wasn't sure about which specific catalyst set off either a physical or thinking challenge, my MS symptoms rarely seemed to go away or appear one at a time.

In the end, solving the question of which MS symptom was more disabling wasn't as important as recognizing that I needed to actually *do something* about my MS. I needed help, and accepting medication deserved serious, immediate consideration.

Tips for Living
Reviewing Options for MS Medication

- ◆ When recommended by a neurologist, consider starting treatment with one of the approved medications to slow the progression of MS. Fortunately, there is a selection.
- ◆ The choice of medication is ultimately up to each patient. However, you should insist on receiving a recommendation from a neurologist as to which medication is best suited for you and your specific symptoms, especially when cognitive issues are a concern.

◆ Compare the materials available from each drug manufacturer and review the options carefully with your support person.

◆ Talk to your neurologist about the possible side effects of your primary medication therapy and any complementary medications you may be using.

Acknowledging MS Cognitive Challenges

◆ Slow down and absorb details. Avoid the compulsion to fill all of your free time with activity. Rest your mind between activities. Take a rest or nap for 15–30 minutes to recharge your mental energy, but avoid sleeping for longer periods during the day, because this can leave you drowsy and irritable.

◆ Reduce or eliminate distractions during conversations and while performing tasks. Turn off the television or radio unless it is useful as background noise.

◆ Ignore the telephone's ring and call-waiting feature. Return calls when you can concentrate.

◆ Have conversations in physical environments where distractions can be kept to a minimum.

◆ Complete one task at a time. A home repair, returning telephone calls, reading, and physical therapy/occupational therapy (PT/OT) exercises can all be accomplished in one day; but allow each task adequate spacing so that two or more activities are not left uncompleted at any one time.

◆ Schedule the most fatiguing work during the times of your highest stamina.

◆ Avoid pushing yourself to the point of fatigue. Step back, take a break, and allow yourself the opportunity to return to the project later, refreshed and more aware of the details involved.

◆ Explain to your immediate family and close friends the ways in which you need to limit your activities. Provide them with a specific schedule as to when you will be available. Sometimes operating with MS limits can be planned; at other times, changes may be dictated by stress and fatigue. Be aware of how your body might malfunction under these circumstances and be prepared to back off from commitments.

◆ Allow family and friends to assist you with endeavors that may unduly tax the limits of your mind and body. Let them know what would be helpful and when you need help. Be honest with yourself and them, permitting yourself to ask for and receive assistance.

◆ Learn to recognize and understand your own anger—not only what situations can light your fuse, but also how to manage MS obstacles so that others do not bear the aftershock of your frustration. Anger about MS is normal, but properly dealing with the effects of MS is the patient's responsibility. Seek professional counseling before it becomes critically necessary.

◆ Remain open to constructive comments and suggestions.

◆ Keep in mind that denying your emotions and avoiding potentially useful changes in your life may be counterproductive.

CHAPTER SIX

The Family Mask

Dr. Matthais's computer musically chimed, noting an incoming e-mail. She didn't flinch at the sound, and her back remained turned away from the screen. Despite having a doctor's typical caseload, she was focused and organized. Her desk was clear of files and loose notes. The wall on the right held her framed diplomas, and on the left were pictures of her husband and children, confirming that it really was her office.

"I'm amazed that you've been able to function as an attorney for this long with MS," she said, "especially with no one detecting your lapses."

"My life feels like a house of cards built on rushing water, and I'm just waiting to either collapse or be pulled under at any moment." Her office was especially warm, and I loosened my tie and released the top button of my starched white shirt. Even sitting motionless in the office chair, my knees felt wobbly and my legs were like melting butter ready to pour down onto the carpet. As I thought about taking off my shoes and socks, I forgot what I had just said. To avoid mild quivering, I held my pen as if I were preparing to write something down on an invisible pad of paper. *What were we talking about?* I wondered.

"How have you made it through the past few months without making a mistake in your work?" said Dr. Matthais.

I had wondered this myself. "I don't think there were any mistakes," I answered, slowly shaking my head from side to side. "Judges and opposing attorneys have a habit of bluntly pointing out those things at the slightest opening."

I had scaled back my office responsibilities and litigation stress, but it wasn't enough to turn down new clients and ask other attorneys in my office to work the cases for me. Although shifting some cases to mediation reduced court time, the heaping mounds of details and intense rounds of negotiations didn't change. Whether I was in court or sitting at a conference room table in my office, I was left absentminded, surrounded by a wall of case files. There was no predictability to my mental lapses. MS didn't work on a schedule. It moved invisibly forward at its own pace.

And then it happened right in front of Dr. Matthais. She was talking, and had asked me a question, I think. The room had become a soft, white fuzz, and I couldn't speak. My eyes were focused on the front of her desk, and without looking up, I could tell that she had leaned forward and was staring at me.

"Are you all right?" she said. My throat swelled with words, but nothing came out. I held my hand up with a "Give me a moment" gesture. My mind floated around, grasping at leftover thoughts about walking into the appointment. There was no hiding it in her office. Right then and there, my ability to think had shut down. We sat quietly for a moment or two.

"I think I'm back," I said. My head was still bent toward the floor. I had definitely drifted away from the conversation. It probably was less than a minute, but when gasping for a mental breath, it was a small eternity.

"Your face was glazed over," said Dr. Matthais. "Was that one of those moments?" As I nodded, my face flushed red with embarrassment. *Better here in a hospital than anywhere else*, I thought.

"Normally, this would be a good time to talk about your aversion to starting medication," said Dr. Matthais, "but I think we'll save that discussion for the next appointment when you're not so disoriented."

We both knew that MS had made its point, and that it would have to be dealt with *sooner* rather than later.

◆　◆　◆

"Daddy, you can walk faster than that," said Lauren, "I'm beating you." This time, I wasn't holding back, pretending she was the speediest walker in the family. She had indeed noticed something during our walk to the store. The more I pressed on, cautiously lifting my legs forward to avoid catching my toes, the more exhausting the effort became.

Of course, Dr. Matthais had been correct to point out that my insistence on hiding my symptoms and avoiding medication was self-defeating. This classic battle to control denial, hiding it from family, sounded like an old echo. Trying to control denial was, in fact, just another form of denial.

During our next appointment, Dr. Matthais turned her attention to why I refused to take medication, even though it was the only possible way to slow progression of the disease. I explained to her how my rejection of medication went beyond resistance to the mixing of medication and self-injecting.

Medication can slow the progression of MS and lessen the severity of symptoms.

"I've been working very hard during the past several years to not bring MS into my house," I said. "This is not like hiding a bottle of pills in the bathroom cabinet. Injecting an MS drug would be a lifestyle change and type of dependency that I don't want my kids to see."

"If you don't start drug therapy, and you allow yourself to become disabled, your girls will certainly see it, but by then it may be too late."

We reviewed how I had been "handling" MS exacerbations at home, and it became clear that I was kidding myself. My struggle with MS may have been disguised, but the disease was affecting Terri and the children. Dr. Matthais was right.

◆ ◆ ◆

"Dr. Lazow never made any sense to me, either, but if both of your doctors now think you should be using one of the drugs," said Terri, "then maybe it's time to start."

I reluctantly nodded my head. Terri did not relish the idea of my taking injections, but she knew that it was time for us to take another look at everything we knew about MS, and for me to accept treatment. Although it was not an easy decision, it was worth another review of the available medications. Even if there wasn't a cure for

MS, taking medication might help more than what I was currently doing—which was nothing.

"Do you still have all of those booklets and videos that Dr. Lazow gave you about the different drugs? I remember looking through at least three different boxes of information and watching the tapes," Terri said, although she already knew how I would answer.

"But it felt so good to throw them in the garbage!" I said, avoiding her eyes. "I really thought I was fine and wouldn't need any of that stuff, so why keep it?" It was a pathetic excuse, equal to a child blaming the dog for eating his homework. Unfortunately, I wasn't 9 years old and we had a cat.

The drug manufacturers' information was easily replaced, but the process of choosing an appropriate MS-fighting medication was daunting. The drugs that I had to choose from nicely followed the alphabet: Avonex®, Betaseron®, and Copaxone®. Terri and I repeatedly watched the videos and read the printed materials, noting their promises, disclaimers, and potential side effects.

Each drug involved injection with needles, but Avonex® was different in two ways. It was injected only once a week, instead of daily or every other day like the other MS medications. (It was a deep, intermuscular shot. *Ouch*, I thought.) More importantly, Avonex® was reported to offer a measured slowing of the progression of *cognitive* symptoms. This was not a cure for MS or a reversal of existing lesions, but rather a chance to slow the development of further cognitive challenges. The fact that Avonex® acknowledged the existence of cognitive problems was encouraging. It offered no guarantees, but it identified and might resist the dual prongs of my symptoms. Avonex® wasn't a threat; it was a tool of action and hope.

MS medications can be tools of action and hope.

However, there would be one condition to my use of this medication. The name *Avonex®* sounded more like a product to clean bathroom tiles than an injectable substance. So I proclaimed that we would call it *Avonéx*, with a silent "x" and pronounced with a slight French accent. This made it sound soft. Even the name of the French MS Society was appealing: Association pour la Recherche sur la Sclérose en Plaques (their Web site looked like a travel brochure). With this emphasis on pronouncing Avonex® with a more continental flare, Terri and I could speak freely about it in public or in front of the children. Others would be left to wonder if we were talking about an exotic type of yoga or a cooking school. Creating a soft name was a way to take part ownership in the medication process.

◆ ◆ ◆

Our front doorbell rang in the middle of a Thursday afternoon, a time when Terri and our girls would not yet be home and my work calendar had been cleared. The home-care nurse, Tracy, stood at our front door wearing a pale-blue nurse's coat. She was here to train me in how to fight MS with injectable medication.

A box of medication and supplies had already been delivered to my office several days earlier, multilabeled with red letters "KEEP REFRIGERATED." Two staff members brought the box to my office with coy smiles on their faces.

"When do we eat?" said Paulette, our curious and hungry recep-tionist. The cord attached to her telephone headset was dangling over her shoulder as she gazed at the chilled package.

"It isn't fresh salmon, chocolates, or any delicacy that you would ever want to eat," I said, taking the box from her hands. Inside the cardboard was an ice-brick chilled Styrofoam container holding four unmixed doses of Avonex®—the first four weeks of medication.

I took it home and stowed the container of supplies and Avonex® out of sight on the bottom shelf of our refrigerator behind a carton of strawberries and a package of cream cheese.

Measuring and mixing the vials of powder with sterile water was easy enough. Following Tracy's instructions, I assembled a practice syringe with a needle and held it as if prepared to throw darts.

"You can practice your injection technique on an orange before you inject your leg," she said. "Injecting an orange is similar to inject-ing into a muscle."

"We have plenty of oranges," I said, "but I'm not sure which one has MS." She smiled, possibly sensing that I was apprehensive about the scene being laid out on our kitchen table. After about 12 jabs into the innocent fruit, I had mastered the quick, smooth forearm/wrist action. My fresh orange bled its juice onto the table without once crying out.

Then it was time for the leg. Without any prompting, I measured and mixed the Avonex®, carefully filling the syringe to the 1.0-cc hash mark. As I cleaned a target area on my right leg with an alcohol wipe, the fumes filled my nostrils, replacing the lingering orange scent. The new needle rivaled the size of an Atlantic whale harpoon, although the nurse would have insisted that it was the same size as the practice needle.

If I had asked her to inject the drug into my thigh, I would never have been able to do it myself. Never. I needed to learn to do this on my own.

"Why don't they have Avonex® pills?" I said, stalling and hoping for another option.

"Some medications can't make it through the digestive system and remain effective," she said.

This was not a happy answer.

> MS often requires continuing to realign priorities, realizing what is truly important

"When you're ready, take a deep breath and inject your leg with the same dart-like rhythm as for the orange," she continued.

It was no different than learning how to slam an industrial steel door on my finger, while telling myself to relax and not move during the process. Hesitation in the injection or jerking my thigh would only make it more painful.

It was now or never for this personal game of Body-Jarts. With a tightly held breath, I plunged the needle into my leg and quickly released my grip of the syringe. When the needle went deep into the muscle, the syringe stood upright from my leg. It looked like a flag planted on another planet. Depressing the plunger and injecting the medication was the easy part.

"Will there be any reaction to the medication?" I said. "Can I go for a run?" Other than wiping a drop of blood from my leg with gauze, I felt no different after removing the needle and tossing it into the protective red container. Feeling energized by successfully completing the procedure, I couldn't wait to get out of the house.

"That's up to you," she said, "but there are typically flu-like symptoms associated with Avonex®. They don't last long and people report that they no longer get them after several months of taking the medication."

MS medications can have varying side effects, but as with other drugs each person's response will be different.

"Do you mean the achy-flu and 'I need chicken soup' side effects?" I said.

"There may be chills and fever, body-aches, and general weakness. That's why most people inject before bedtime—so they can sleep through the initial discomfort. The Tylenol® that I asked you to take before we started should help reduce side effects."

Later, as I ran along the Lake Park pathway, I felt a twinge in my leg where the medication had been injected. Despite the dull ache and feeling overheated, I extended my legs out further to cover more ground, quickly exhausting my stamina. The comparison to an attempt to outrun the disease was obvious, but I had to stop after running only 1 mile. As my body began to tremble under the strain of standing up, I decided to slowly wobble home.

Later, I was awakened in the middle of the night by the quivering of the bed. My body was uncontrollably shaking and I felt cold, yet sweated out. The side effects had arrived.

"Can I get you anything?" said Terri.

"The Tylenol® wore off," I mumbled into the darkness.

"How about another blanket and some more Tylenol®?" she said, rubbing my quivering shoulder gently.

The nurse had said that the side effects would only last for about 24 hours and should diminish over several months. Although this wasn't immediately comforting, I had to trust that the discomforts would be temporary. It was never pleasant, but my particular "flu" would dependably come and go within 36 hours, and there was always peace in sleeping through it.

The first several weeks of injecting the drug were filled with periods of hesitation and lack of confidence. The loaded syringe would be clenched in my hand, sometimes for 20 or 30 minutes, but adding more time to the routine did not translate into having the nerve to inject the needle into my leg. After about 6 weekly injections, however, a routine emerged. It was a step-by-step process that included clearing the table, laying out the unmixed medication and supplies, lighting a candle, watching *Frasier* on TV, and grinding the evening coffee. Somewhere in that quiet, calm, lock-step process there was an injection. The jab was surrounded by soft and distracting points of routine.

With the exception of Terri and my doctors, no one knew about my use of Avonex®, including our children. Anticipation of the injections was like a cold bucket of ice water down my back. It was unwelcome, yet it was also empowering.

Accepting medication for MS can be empowering.

Acceptance of MS was not easy, and I dreaded the needles. However, it now felt more like I was confronting MS, rather than skillfully denying it. When I pounded the empty syringe into the red Sharps container, there was more than just relief at completing the shot. It was a push back against the disease. I was doing something about my MS, not simply waiting for it to steal the feeling in my limbs and obscure my thoughts. Despite my worst apprehension, I was fighting the MS in my body.

◆ ◆ ◆

People were starting to notice something was different about me. While on a vacation weekend at the lake with friends, someone asked why I was walking "a little funny." During the Purim carnival at my synagogue, my legs went out from under me and I fell. One of the other volunteers stared at me, as if stunned to see me lying on the floor. My speedskating coach commented, "Your straightaways are as good as ever, but you don't hold the corners anymore."

One warm June evening, I loaded the girls into their red wagon and headed in the direction of the ice cream store. Later, I told Dr. Matthais, "I pulled the wagon only with my right arm to protect and hide my limp. It was a good *Hunchback of Notre Dame* rhythm, and the necessary pauses were concealed by counting the kitties and puppies crossing our path."

Dr. Matthais looked stunned at the idiocy of the male ego. "If you are having problems standing and walking, and pulling the wagon hurts your arm, why didn't you just let your wife pull it?"

I was challenged by her simple question, but could only envision my children's reaction. The room was silent, and then I said "Because I'm *Daddy!*" This defensive explanation was shortened by my need to suppress the sudden choke in my voice. As her eyes welled up, Dr. Matthais shifted her gaze to the framed photos of her own young children displayed on the bookcase. "If you start crying, then I'll be joining you," I said. This was not about sentiment, but my comment had touched a family chord for both of us.

"Even with the Avonex®, I still don't want our kids to know about my MS. I intended to play the illusion of physically active Daddy for as long as possible."

"Don't be too sure that they haven't seen it already," said Dr. Matthais.

Deep down, I knew she was right.

The numbness in my leg was pronounced. The sensation of walking on anesthetized nerves filled the leg, as it had previously done with my hand, face, and skull. The leg was heavy, and it maneuvered awkwardly, even on the straightaways. Finally, when my walking buckled while crossing a bus-filled street near our home, I accepted Dr. Thomas's recommendation to try IV steroids. Arguing against a week of hospitalization, I asked him if I could be treated at home under the watchful eyes of a visiting nurse.

"If you can be quiet and physically inactive for the duration," said Dr. Thomas, "then we can arrange to do this at home. Since there will be an IV line inserted into a vein, it is important that you keep the arm still and not dislodge the line." It sounded horrible, but it was still better than staying in the hospital for a week, away from Terri and our girls.

So, we turned the guest room into an outpatient clinic filled with IV stands, boxes of syringes, needles, tubes, flushing saline, and medication drip bags. Terri and I shielded this room and the visiting home-care nurse from our children, but I was no longer hiding from MS. Now, I was actually doing something about it—fighting back.

Steroid medication can be used short term to bring symptoms under control.

I never felt alone when I stepped into the room and closed the door for a couple hours. Terri's support was always present on either side of the door—whether it was arranging the tubes and clamps, or plunging connectors into the different liquid bags. The children playing upstairs could be heard throughout the house, and whenever the sounds of small footsteps approached the closed door, Terri was there to redirect their attention to another activity—away from the "hospital" room. Seeing Daddy plugged into a hanging drip-bag, surrounded by IV supplies scattered across the bed and desk, would have been a curious shock for our daughters.

Watching the slow-drip of the IV had a hypnotic effect, and I measured my own breathing against the timed speed of each steroid drop—not too fast or too slow. As the clear fluid seeped into my vein, I felt a cool rush from the chill of the room-temperature solution. The core of my forearm felt like it was being slowly submerged into a pool of glacier water. My overheated body was being air-conditioned from the inside out.

"Did you sleep any better last night?" said Terri. She had entered the kitchen and noticed that I had already finished an early morning breakfast. "Your eyes are red."

The potent steroids flowing through my system had the nightly effect of taping my eyelids open and shifting my brain into a previously unknown sixth gear. There wasn't a single moment of sleep, not even a slight doze. The stunning 23-hour awareness was way beyond the experience of oral steroids.

"Did we accidentally switch the IV and espresso bags?" I said. "No wonder the stuff is illegal for professional athletes. Since I was up the whole night, I used the time to mentally rearrange and paint the basement. Tonight, I'll work on closets and spring plantings for the backyard."

"Should we call Dr. Thomas?" said Terri. "You need to be able to sleep, sometime."

"There's probably little we can do about it until I'm finished with the treatment. Besides, I would hate to take more medication to help with the steroids, which are bolstering the Avonex®—drugs to help the drugs that are helping the drugs." We both smiled at my ridiculous explanation. "Just don't let me use this arm, and it'll be over soon enough."

◆ ◆ ◆

The glacier hiking trails of the Kettle-Moraine area had the sound of coolness, but I hesitated at the thought of a long walk. It was a pre-arranged hike through ravines and unpaved woods with several other families we had known for years. It didn't matter that I had been dragging all day, avoiding unnecessary trips up and down the stairs at home. Since everyone else was going on the jaunt, then we were all going, too. If covering up drop-foot by blaming uneven cement was good masking and somewhat logical, then falling down into a root-and-stone-strewn valley might not be too suspicious.

The Sunday morning sun sliced through the living room blinds covering Lauren and Meredith, who were sitting on the hardwood floor. They were putting on warm socks, hoping to block the brisk winds along the trail. Looking down at the treads of my dark leather Timberline shoes, I recalled Dr. Thomas's suggestion that I consider being fitted for an orthopedic foot brace, but I let the notion slide. It was time to get in the car and far too late for regrets.

"You're bringing it?" said Terri, pointing at the wooden walking cane I clutched in my hand.

"It seems like a good time to use it, don't you think?"

"I'm not saying 'Don't'. But I've never seen you use it in front of anyone before."

Up to that point, I had thought there was a *mask* for every MS occasion, but hiding in the open was delicate.

As we pulled into the stone-covered parking lot, I noticed that our group of about 30 adults and children was gathering at the edge of the woods.

"Daddy," said Meredith, "I'll get your stick!" As she reached down to the floor mat to grab the cane, I stepped out of the car.

"Leave it," I said. "Everyone just hang here for a minute, and I'll be right back." I turned from three curious faces and hobbled off into an adjacent clump of trees. Within a few minutes, I returned to the car carrying three large sticks, which I had broken down to size from fallen branches.

"Now we all have walking sticks for the hike," said Terri. Under-standing my scheme, she smiled and grabbed the taller of the sticks, while I handed the small ones to the girls. With the slight exception that my "stick" was varnished and had a black rubber stopper on the tip, it all blended together. What looked like a family hike was actually a *family mask*, a disguise covering my stumbling leg and MS. Perhaps it was a clever moment, but it was not a long-term answer.

Eventually, everyone would learn about my MS, but since I couldn't imagine a graceful way to impart the diagnosis, I chose to say nothing during the group hike. The conversation disclosing my MS was neither casual nor fulfilling, unlike talking openly about expecting a baby or a new job would have been. MS couldn't be covered during the typical greeting exchange of "How are you?" permitting the response of "Fine, how are you?" Whether it would be "early retirement" or "chronic, progressive, disabling neurological disease," the honesty of the words would never be easy.

◆ ◆ ◆

Painkillers can be used to lessen the side effects of MS medication.

After 10 months of injections, the side effects had not subsided. They didn't get worse, but they certainly didn't diminish, as the training nurse had suggested they would.

"Our records show that you have been using Avonex® for almost a year," said the pharmacist for Biogen, the manufacturer of the medication. "There are a small percentage of patients who continue to have flu-like symptoms beyond the normal four- to six-month period, about 10 to 15 percent."

"Great," I said, "now I'm part of another *special* group."

"You may wish to speak to your neurologist. Prescriptions for stronger painkillers can be taken just prior to injections. This should help get you through the first 24 hours."

There was no way to know for sure whether the Avonex® was slowing down the course of my MS. However, I was well past the point of remaining idle, watching and waiting for the next numbing exacerbation. *Stay the course,* I repeatedly told myself. *Try to find ways of making the injection process easier, less intimidating, and more routine.* The Biogen folks were always willing to provide support and training if I needed it. They sent extra gauze, alcohol wipes, and even a jazz CD to ease my mind. Relaxing remained a priority, equal to avoiding overheating and fatigue.

The training nurse was not there to inject me on a weekly basis, so I had to rely on myself, creating a personal commitment to the treatment. My acceptance of medication was bolstered by the many reasons to pursue its possible benefits. It was my best chance of stopping further growth of my MS lesions, so that when a *cure* became available, my mind and limbs would not be too far gone.

The monthly shipments of Avonex® were preserved by an ice block until they were placed in the refrigerator. We had also stored several of the blocks in our freezer for use later in our picnic cooler. The frozen blocks sustained the potent medication, but they also helped my legs. Once the injection target site had been selected, I would press the frozen block onto the spot and hold it down firmly with a thick cloth under my fingertips. After about 10 minutes, the area below the skin would be numb from the cold, making the injection less painful.

For some people, self-injecting medication may be nothing more than a small aggravation, like taking out the garbage. I wasn't at that point, yet, and I kept looking for possible ways to make the process easier. I asked Dr. Thomas if a shorter, thinner needle would still be effective, and he agreed to prescribe one. "A one-inch, 25-gauge needle should still get the medication deep enough into the muscle," he said. "Try it and see if it feels any better."

It sounded so simple. The shorter, thinner needle meant less pain, affording the best chance that I wouldn't become discouraged. These were small, yet meaningful changes to the injection protocol, but they worked to lessen my anticipation of the shot, which in truth was far worse than the shot itself. These simple ways of owning the injection process bolstered my decision to continue taking the MS medication.

Nothing stopped the tremors that sometimes took over my hands, causing my fingers to uncontrollably shake the syringe in my grasp—not deep breathing exercises, soft music, or peaceful thoughts.

"Is there any way I can help with injections?" said Terri. "You seem so frustrated."

"I can steady my hands on the table while mixing the medication, and push the medication in while my arm rests on my leg. But with these tremors, I've lost accuracy in holding the angle and hitting the right spot deep enough."

"I'll do that part," she said. Then she took the needle from my shaking hand, counted to three, and plunged it into my leg. Next, she let go of the syringe and jerked back. She had hit the mark perfectly, and we both stared at the planted syringe and sighed with relief.

"Always remember," I said, "this hurts me more than it hurts you."

She shook her head as if trying to release herself from the moment.

"Do you know how many people would love to have the regular opportunity to jab their spouses?" I teased.

"Not like this," she responded.

I was comfortable with this change to my night injection maneuvers. Terri had really come through for me just when the routine of treatment was at risk. Given the opportunity to join my battle against MS, people often surprise me with their willingness to get involved— if I could only take off the mask and let them.

◆ ◆ ◆

After months of fighting, I knew it was finally time to let go of my career as a lawyer. Nothing seemed changed as I drove to the office, prepared to make "the announcement." But after finishing the morning staff greetings and checking messages, everything did change. With only a few minutes' notice, I had assembled the entire staff and announced that I had MS and was retiring from the practice of law. Then I walked out of the conference room and away from their stunned silence. I didn't know where to go or what to do next. I was casting off with no destination in sight. It had been almost 5 years since my initial diagnosis.

Back in my office with the door closed, I faced a stack of my medical records and the disability forms that I needed to fill out. I pictured myself leaping into a rowboat moored on a wide and unfamiliar coastline. A thick fog has rolled in and dusk has fallen. I am pushed off toward a rumored safe harbor and have been instructed to "leave it all behind, keep rowing, and wait for a landfall." After months of rowing, there are still no landmarks to corroborate the proper direction. My family is waiting for me, counting on me.

Off in the distance, I hear the rolling echo of a storm headed toward me. It is impossible to know whether I will reach land before the storm takes me under. All I can do is just keep rowing toward the perceived shore.

The notice in the mail was simple: the Social Security Department of the United States Government had decided that I was a disabled person. Although it had previously been confirmed by neurologists and a top-level insurance company, the letter was a shock. It seemed so final.

I had arrived into retirement with a quiet thump, like Dorothy in the Land of Oz. Terri was teaching in her classroom; our girls were at school. At home, it was just me and Mickey, the cat, staring at recently delivered boxes of legal books and a stack of framed prints that had formerly hung on my office walls.

Working through the list of household chores didn't fill the missing career void or provide a sense of accomplishment, and I doubted that I would ever feel comfortable kicking back and doing nothing. My Grandpa Harry used to say that you must be active in retirement, because you can only take out the garbage once a day. He worked until his death at the age of 96. But I was now only 41 years old.

MS often requires a continuing realignment of priorities.

At first, the news about my retirement and MS spread slowly. There were sympathetic hugs when I least expected them from a friend or neighbor. Soon the news about my health took off, catching me off guard in conversations but saving me the awkwardness of having to bring up the subject. Handshakes turned into supportive embraces, breaking the barrier of my formal, attorney attitude. The understanding and support was meant for me and my family. It was not perfunctory, but rather it was as if each person was imparting resolve and strength to help us cope with my symptoms and confront the disease.

> Help yourself to be stronger by helping others. Volunteering is often more valuable to the volunteer than to the recipient of the assistance.

Filling a space as large as a career shouldn't be difficult. The trick is to ensure that it isn't filled with meaningless, time-consuming activities. Unless something of substance replaced my career and State Bar interests, my time could easily be taken up with the well-intended suggestions of others:

"As long as you have the time, why don't you volunteer to take over the Temple's Bingo nights?" said one congregant.

"The automobile dealer's association is looking for volunteer arbitrators to decide car purchase disputes," offered another friend. Although being asked to join the board of directors for a local nursing home might sound like a simple volunteering invitation, it might also bring with it a new briefcase full of stress.

Although I appreciated the diverse suggestions, I wanted to do more than simply fill in my emptied sandpit with different-colored sand. The decisions boiled down to core questions: What is really vital to pursue without being detrimental to my health and the well-being of my family? Do I have the burning drive to pursue a particular mission? If the answer is "no" to either of these questions, it is far better to kindly pass on the opportunity. Every activity had an energy price to pay, and I was careful about whether to jump into anything, whether it was for social action or to paint a room in the house. My limits were variable and uncertain.

> The manufacturers of MS medications have many useful educational resources, including Web sites and support hotlines. Don't be left wondering about MS, seek them out to answer your questions.

It didn't matter how well I had masked my MS symptoms from coworkers, family, and friends. There is no awarded medallion for disguising a chronic disease; no gold-plated wheelchair for being able to stand without leaning on something; no Nobel Prize for polishing and lining up all of your mental marbles. I was more than just my legal career and far more than the MS that enveloped me.

Removing the mask and stepping openly into retirement brought peaceful relief and allowed me to see more clearly how to face the disease. In the final analysis, privately maintaining my well-guarded, private world of progressive disability would have only one winner: MS. With medication in my system and a striking realignment of my priorities, maybe I could reach a tolerable plateau.

Tips for Living

Removing the Mask

- Masking and ignoring the symptoms of MS can allow potentially irreparable damage to your health.
- Taking medication for MS is not giving into the disease—it can protect your body from further damage. Use it to buy time until a better medication or cure is found.
- Maintaining your prescribed MS therapy is keeping the promise to yourself and your family that you will fight MS.
- Own the process of injecting medication by making yourself comfortable during the procedure. Ask for help with injections, if necessary.
- Focus your attention on raising your spirit and strength to face new challenges and overcome them, rather than blaming yourself for having MS.
- Stress may cause exacerbations of MS. Limit the stress in your life.
- Limit your commitments to those people and activities that are the most important to you.

Facing Retirement

- Retirement can mean new goals of personal passion and fulfilling purpose.
- Maintain all insurance coverage and review options to immediately maximize your benefits.
- When considering your doctor's recommendation to retire, obtain a copy of your available private and group disability insurance policies, as well as applications for Social Security Disability. Before resigning from any employment—thereby potentially terminating all of your life, disability, and health insurance coverage—investigate your rights regarding benefits.

◆ If you have questions about disability insurance coverage and the application forms, consider seeking immediate legal representation prior to submitting any forms.

◆ Know your legal rights and pursue them with skilled assistance.

CHAPTER SEVEN

Feeling the Edges

Time may heal a lot of things, but apparently not MS brain lesions. Embracing the fact that I am losing control of my mind and body stuck like a piece of sandpaper in my throat and I didn't want to get used to it, even in retirement.

> Cognitive challenges will not be solved with silence. There needs to be broad mainstream discussions of how to face the cognitive challenges of MS.

Overnight I needed to accept that my litigation career was finished. The diplomas would pile up in a drawer and eventually be lost under other outdated papers. My schedule had been wiped clear of appointments and court appearances were moved to an associate's calendar. Through the sheer force of habit, I still got up the next morning and faced the same suits and ties, then stepped into the normal routine like getting gasoline for the car, going to the office, and stopping for bread on the way home. Only two of the three stops were still useful to me.

It felt like I had been to a funeral, as I stepped into the movement of the day and no one knew that a part of me was gone. While nothing around me had changed, it all seemed temporary—like a stage show. With MS in the forefront of my thoughts, it was difficult for me to find a reason to smile and I wondered whether being happy would also be a thing of the past. Despite pretending that I could ditch MS in the pile of my daily tasks, I knew that the road had been yanked out from under my life, leaving me sitting on the curb without clear road signs, the ability to walk far or conceive of a direction. Every step seemed like a wrong move and doing nothing left me at the mercy of more lesions.

As a young boy, I rode my bicycle to Grantosa Drive, a crossroad adjacent to my childhood home on 91st Street and as it cleared the first stoplight, it rolled down into a steep decline for several blocks. It was a favorite road of mine and I could time the green light, after building up a head of steam on my bike and fly across the intersection into a catapulted acceleration. Like an arrow shot out of its bow, I would release my feet from the pedals and hold my legs straight back, *flying* parallel to the ground. With my stomach resting flat on the seat, I could look down and see the tires of my red Schwinn eat up the pavement, while my hair flew up and back with the wind. It seemed effortless in motion and the bike was self-propelled. Coasting was an imaginary blast of power and seemed to be the best way to ride, but had its limits.

Being mentally and physically shredded by brain lesions, there would be no coasting through the MS. The words "multiple sclerosis" were still new for me, but it was clear that there would be no gliding through life, especially now that I have been told that MS is twice the chronic disease that I had earlier anticipated. What are the limits for me and how am I supposed to balance the need to monitor unpredictable physical symptoms with an erratic loss of thinking concepts and vanishing awareness? Last week it was a struggle to remember client names and legal strategies for dozens of cases and now I don't really feel competent to deal with just one minor thing at a time, much less balance two burning health demands.

> Cognitive difficulties may interfere with multitasking, limiting attention and awareness.

When I was 12 years old, my family and I went to the circus where I noticed a young man riding a unicycle and alternately tossing five rings high in the air. While the crowd was amused by his juggling talents, along with his ability to catch a flung hat on his head, I remained focused on the solo wheel of the unicycle. It was the key to his balance and as long as he kept moving, he handled whatever was thrown at him. He never stopped pedaling. There were no gears to shift or any handlebars, brakes, or ability to coast in a neutral gear. If he stopped moving, then he would crash to the ground, followed by the rings. No coasting meant it was more challenging, but not impossible.

It took me most of that summer to master riding the first unicycle that my parents bought for me. The life lesson revealed itself to me again when I was diagnosed with MS and later learned that my thinking had been short-circuited. I had been left to peddle through MS and juggle its multiple cognitive and physical rings. No downhill coasting was allowed and I had to find a way to keep myself moving or crash. There would be no clear map of what I would experience with MS, except anticipating that the destination was a level of disability. There seemed little to do on my own, except maintain my exercise workout and try to keep my body and mind moving ahead of MS.

◆ ◆ ◆

My court schedule had been cleared indefinitely, and after taking some time off of speedskating, I yearned to go back to the ice. If I didn't continue to move my body, I was concerned that it might get used to the idleness. My leg didn't seem ready to return to speedskating, even after receiving rounds of steroids that were probably illegal for competitors. Without the drugs, ice speedskating was a perfect match for MS, since the cold-filtered air maintained my core body temperature at a crisp frost level. Visitors complain that they are freezing, but it is ice, and the colder it is, the better for speedskating.

My running shoes were of little use to me now, since running quickly overheated my body, turning my legs into wet noodles and staggering my balance. My troubled stride wasn't powerful or graceful and a bit scary to experience. Hitting the ground or a tree was likely and for my own safety, along with requests from Terri, I removed myself from the running zone. Fortunately for me, there was still the ice and I was grateful that I had acquired speedskating skills before MS threw road salt in my way. However, I would need the use of both legs.

Ice size does matter and the Pettit Olympic oval dwarfed the two separate hockey rinks placed in the center of the endless loop. Coats and snow boots were replaced by a hooded full-body racing "skin," streamlined sunglasses, and tautly lashed Viking blades. When coming out of a curve, my visual focus was immediately fixed on the distant approaching red pads lining the inside and outside edges of the ice. My mind focused on shifting my whole body weight alternately to balance on the thin blades, as they each sliced forward in line with the straight gaze of my eyes. The oval ice cut through tension and distractions, but most of all, it was my escape from MS.

The three frozen solid lanes provided my body with the exercise that stretched my legs and honed my equilibrium, while sharpening my focus on the technique of gliding on the flat ice and feeling the edges of my blades. The agonizing sense of losing my abilities to track litigation was an energy spike for lapping the oval ice. If the adrenaline fumes from having my career torn away could be a substance for athletic performance enhancement, then its use would be illegal.

But when I couldn't feel my lower left leg being connected to my foot, my balance began to shake. The deadening weakness extended up into my thigh, straining the muscles to carry my weight with equal balance. My knee felt as though it was only attached to a wood stilt and not a calf muscle, foot, and five toes. I might have noticed earlier that some of the sensation in my left foot and toes was lost, except that I lash the skates so tight to my feet that some loss of circulation is normal. For a tight fit, speedskaters don't wear socks, but I knew that wasn't the cause of the problem. My coach, Bob Fenn, had noticed the difficulties that I brought to the ice. I needed to be honest with him and MS.

"If you don't occasionally fall," said Bob, "then you are not trying hard enough!" Bob learned by coaching others to Olympic Gold, and he believed that if speedskating was easy, then everyone would do it. But it isn't and they don't. "Five more laps!" he yelled at our group of speedskaters as we passed by him like a long winding subway train. I was in the middle of the pack and grateful for the dynamic vacuum suction pulling me along. I didn't feel safe and pulled out of the pack. When Bob yells at you, it means that he is paying attention to your technique. Mine was failing and running out of coordination.

"Now cross over again, again!" Bob screamed at me as I stood and glided through the back half of the curve on the ice. He was waiting for me as I cleared the second curve and headed for his coaching "corner" of the oval. Crouching low, while crossing over, can take down Olympians and I wondered why I was still on the ice when my lower left leg was numb. The speed of impact from cross-over crashes has sent speedskaters to the hospital. Even with that thought in mind, I laced up my skates, despite not being able to feel the grip of my toes.

"You pulled out early," said Bob. "We have another twenty minutes, are you done already?"

"Something in me is not working right," I answered. Bob didn't argue with me, which meant that he saw that my glide was off and that something was wrong. Saying nothing to him could lead him to think that I didn't take his coaching seriously or that he was doing something wrong. It was MS on my ice. My left foot couldn't feel the chill of the ice, although no one could tell by just looking at it. My coach deserved to learn the truth and so I told him about my MS diagnosis and numbness.

"I'm sorry for pushing you," said Bob, "I never knew." His voice had softened and his face was heartening, as he coasted by my side down the outer lane. "You just keep as low as you can and don't give up on it," said Bob, pointing out at the ice. His hand rested on my left shoulder, as we drifted down the back straightaway and were lapped by his skaters. "I wish their lazy asses would ride as low as you normally do," he continued, critically watching them as they passed us. Somewhere in there was a compliment.

"Don't you dare let up on me," I said. "I'd notice the silence." It is the only yelling that I appreciated hearing.

> Be prepared to re-evaluate your exercise routine to learn new techniques to be active and safe. Don't give up.

The season ended and so did my competitive skating. My ability to speedskate had changed in the blink of my eyes. With an honest MS explanation, I knew that Bob would do anything possible to make changes in my ice routine, if it would help me to be safe and hold my edges. This was my smoldering incentive to take care of myself and prepare to return to the ice someday.

◆ ◆ ◆

How old am I? It was a potentially disastrous situation, not faced by me since I was 3 years old. There were new limits on what my body would sustain and I needed to identify them. Humiliation from a potential physical letdown would be as humbling as when I collapsed at a truck stop.

The annual United Performing Arts Fund (UPAF) Ride-for-the-Arts raised desperately needed revenue for the arts community in the greater Milwaukee area. Tens of thousands of pledge-filled bicyclists were launched from downtown Milwaukee on various routes across the city. As a member of the UPAF Board of Directors, I volunteered to drive the pace car for the longest route in excess of 25 miles. When I was led to the silver Volkswagen Golf, a convertible pace car, I could smell the new black leather seats before I could see them. Magnetic plaques and brightly colored flags were attached to the doors, along with flashing hazard lights that everyone in the city would be able to see a mile away. Although that was the point of a pace car, I would soon regret the attention. A Channel 4 (NBC) helicopter hovered above us, waiting to catch the start of the ride and film the sea of bicyclists following me down the vacated downtown streets.

This would be *beyond cool*.

A police officer reviewed the UPAF ride map with me, which laid out a looping route through the far south side of Milwaukee. With the radio cranked and the morning sun on my shoulders, I only needed to stay the course safely ahead of the enormous pack of riders. They weren't speedskaters, so there would be no drafting on my pace car. Side streets were blockaded by motorcycle police, squad cars, and barricades, ensuring that I was the only moving motor vehicle on the road, along with thousands of my two-wheeled friends.

I had a light breakfast early that morning. One egg bagel with strawberry cream cheese, a glass of orange juice, two cups of coffee for the caffeine hit, and a precautionary bathroom stop at home.

After clicking the seat belt and receiving last-minute instructions, the path in front of me was cleared of reporters and television cameras. In front of my bumper was the white starting and finishing line—painted across the street. I waited for the signal and thought "no." Not now, not here, please, "no." Where was the warning hint? There should be nothing so immediate. With the cruise control locked at 25 mph, I tightly pinched my legs and followed the open path.

The whirl from the helicopter blades slowly faded, but the rear- and both side-view mirrors were filled with thousands of riders. After several miles I could see a McDonald's restaurant in the distance and I accelerated a two-block distance ahead of the following herd. Perhaps sensing a challenge on the fundraiser ride, several of the lead riders began to stand up on their pedals to crank leverage for speed. I needed space to time a bathroom break and not a car race with bicycles.

Although I could punch the accelerator into the parking lot and quickly pass through the restaurant's bathroom, they would catch up with me within a minute or less. I am not that fast even in the woods and they were approaching like a wild stampede of caribou. If I stopped, then the restaurant and my pace car would be encased with the pandemonium of thousands of bicycles at an unmarked stop, swarming and waiting for direction and pacing. There would be no simple escape and the convertible would be caught like a dolphin in a tuna net.

Turning off the cruise control, I slowed the car and watched the oasis restaurant pass by as I scanned ahead for the turnaround checkpoint. Tall trees and low cropped bushes lined the streets—so no help there. As I approached the circular turnaround point, my eyes were fixed on the bathroom line, which was already ten deep and surrounded by tables with hundreds of filled water cups. Neither sight was helpful to my predicament. And they were still following me!

Previously, when I attended one of the NMSS Newly Diagnosed Series for MS persons and their caregivers, I noticed a brochure on the information table that dealt with bladder control or resulting accidents. The cover noted a feature article about proper diet and exercises to maintain independence and other promises of liberty. The common-sense advice was for everyone and I figured it might be of interest to me in twenty-five years. Since I was still in my thirties, I presumed that information must be for others. Maybe I should have taken that brochure home for a glance.

> Check with the NMSS and other respected MS organizations and take note of their (free) publications and brochures. Be open to learning more about how MS may affect you now and in the future. The information may be frightening at first, but it is best to know all you can and know all of your options.

Presuming that the riders would know how to retrace their marked path and that my role was finished, I slowly turned the flashing convertible through the parking lot and began the torturous trek toward the downtown starting point. I floored it, silently praying to the kindergarten potty-god for groin clamping endurance. There was no way, absolutely no way I would make it without a car accident—I mean an accident in the car. But this was not the type of car "accident" that I feared, glancing at the supple black leather seats. Ditching the car into the Milwaukee River seemed like a far more reasonable course of action than making a small puddle on the European styling. Turning away from the river, I decided against a morning UPAF swim.

It was not my colorful flag streaming car, so I drove it up the curb near the finishing line and parked it on the sidewalk adjacent to the blue line of portable bathrooms—just in time. Even driving a pace car, I learned that MS could reach for me at its discretion and even overtake me. I needed to prepare myself much better than this and accept the available MS educational materials, learning from the practical experiences of others, before they happened to me.

◆ ◆ ◆

The combination of Disney, Hollywood, and television comedian Bernie Mac was coming to town to make a baseball movie, *Mr. 3000*. If I could withstand the hours of boredom as an official movie "extra," then maybe I could use the sitting time to sort through some of the MS materials that I had received from the NMSS. Being retired, I also needed something fun to do, I figured. I stuffed a couple of MS books, brochures and a legal pad of paper in my backpack as I headed to the first night's filming at our new baseball stadium, Miller Park. Jotting down private MS thoughts and concerns became a sincere and open window into my grappling with the new rules for my life.

Changes had arrived, but please get me away from the talk about multiple brain lesions, MRIs, hospital waiting rooms, medication with needles, blood tests, numbness, losing my memories, and problem-solving skills. Just let me disappear into a crowd of extras, pretending that we are sitting at a stadium watching a real sporting event, without a trace of identity or discussion of my MS. People in Hollywood change their names, faces, and personas all the time, so I and the MS should be invisible under the camera lights. Right?

Bernie Mac was portraying a major league baseball player with the Milwaukee Brewers who would retire immediately after his 3,000th hit. I was directed to sit in an area along the first-base line where Bernie's 3,000th hit would be tossed into our group of extras. We didn't have the script and weren't told what Bernie's character would do, but we understood that he would personally come after the ball in the middle of the game and claim it for himself. It was a critical moment in the movie plot and I held a camera that was given to me as a prop, "acting" like I was taking photos of the historic 3,000th hit. The ball was tossed and caught several seats to my right. I remained by my seat on the aisle, acting like I was a typical fan taking pictures of the moment, but the scene didn't end with the catch.

Without warning, Bernie Mac continued past first base and headed to leave the field in the midst of play and marched toward our group of standing extras. Off camera, he normally approached us with a wide smile and a few jokes, but this time he was fuming and humorless.

"Open the gate!" Bernie yelled to the gate usher. "Open the gate!" The acting usher was confused by why Bernie, a "player," would try to enter the stands during a game, even if it was just a movie. We were supposed to leap to our feet as the ball was hit toward us, but my left leg was numb and it didn't care that it was in a movie. I pulled on the seat in front of me to yank myself up and hobbled into the aisle near the gate while clicking photos like several other extras. The railing supported me as I continued to watch through the viewfinder. Bernie Mac flung the gate open and stomped into the aisle, steaming furiously like a steer leading the running of the bulls.

"Who's got the damn ball?" he shouted at our group. "Who's got the damn ball?!" With his storming face now filling the viewfinder of my camera, I snapped another photo and was glad that he had dropped the bat on the field.

"Is this part of the movie?" I asked another extra, who was cowering next to me in the raging path of Bernie Mac. The movie cameras continued to roll without anyone calling "Cut." Bernie was scanning the area where the ball would have landed and kept marching up the aisle toward me. If he wanted the precious baseball, then I figured that he would turn into one of the rows of extras in front of me to retrieve it. Bernie moved up the aisle stairs like a wild animal close to a kill. I was still leaning against the railing for stability when he approached, then looked toward the caught ball and forearmed us out of the way. My right leg moved backward to catch the push, but my left leg didn't follow and caused me to stumble backward. My right leg took an extra hop before I tumbled down hard against a cement step behind me. Another Extra tripped over me and crashed down on my legs. We stared at each other in amazement as the crowd pressed in around us.

"Cut, cut, cut," yelled Doug, the Paramount director of the scene. Bernie had stopped lunging forward and turned toward our film-stopping commotion. He leaned in over me, smiling in amusement of how the scene unfolded.

"I told you I'd kick your ass!" said Bernie, as he hovered over us and began laughing at our tumbled faces. Although I tried to sit up, I couldn't get my left leg to move under me. Invisible arms gently lifted me to my feet and braced me until I could grab the railing. My body felt like a stuntman trampled by the buffalo in *Dances with Wolves*. One of the film crew, Steve, saw the fall and called me over to his recording equipment.

"I thought it was you who crashed," said Steve. "We saw it happen on our monitors and then the crowd swarmed in and we lost sight of you. Are you all right?"

"Minor bruises," I answered. Bernie may have given me an arm push to move me away, but I knew that it was my MS that caused the trip to the cement. Even the script of a Hollywood film couldn't provide an escape from MS. Blending into a crowd of extras, my MS was still noticeable and ignoring it injured me. I had purchased a cane and deliberately left it at home, thinking that my MS would stand out with a cane in hand. The learned truth was that I didn't avoid unwanted attention by crashing to the concrete ground. Maybe MS wouldn't be as troublesome if I was more braced for its impact.

> Accept an assistive device when available. Your safety and mobility are paramount to independence.

A few short years later I learned that Bernie Mac had died at the age of 50. I found myself holding the baseball that he had signed for me. Life moves away too fast and I realized that I need to acknowledge the numerous and unwanted changes in my life before they overtake me. Whether it would be on the ice, on film, or just pacing out a long car ride, I would need to better understand MS and continue to accept help while learning to deal with the unpredictable change-up. I held the baseball tight in my grip.

◆ ◆ ◆

What would I lose next that I wouldn't perceive? Retiring didn't mean that I would also leave the MS behind me, since the mental and physical stumbling would certainly follow me. Although the physical challenges were visible and more apparent, the cognitive losses were imperceptible until there was a noted mental void. I couldn't help but wonder about the missing pieces, perhaps a vital detail from our checking account or family and home concerns. Tax returns, I won't even go there. The mental self-doubt list was growing as pieces of my essence were left aside. Like emptying ballast from a ship taking on water, I felt as though MS would jettison the reliable memories of my life. Was it reasonable to wonder about the end point and what segments of my mind and body would remain?

When I get on an airplane, I like to know where it is headed and learn about what to expect when I get there. So far, reading the glossy magazine stuffed in the seat pocket in front of me, I am not looking forward to reaching this final destination. Am I just another MS passenger or do I have the ability to direct the course of this vehicle? My seat belt is connected, just in case.

Tips for Living

◆ When the basics in your life are changing, then discover what is now open to you, rather than be overly concerned about what may be lost. Consider retiring on your terms and focus on taking your passions and interests to a new level.

◆ Allow yourself to be totally distracted by the good things in your life. Relish the moments of doing things to remind yourself that you are alive. Discover entertaining and challenging experiences. Many more amazing moments lie ahead for you. Don't give up on yourself and keep it interesting.

◆ Redefine your physical exercises and cognitive activities to keep fit and active. Look for ways to hold on to what you enjoy. Stay strong.

◆ Review the NMSS catalog of topics, including the direction of MS research studies. Don't be afraid of the information. MS is not the same for everyone. Even though many of the MS subtopics in these materials may not currently apply to you, plant a seed in your mental MS library and know that on-point information is ready if and when you need it. Consider it to be your private archive of MS maps and life strategies.

◆ If you would like others to understand your MS limits and sometimes lend assistance, then share with them how they may specifically help you. Careful on the ice and grab a hand when needed for balance.

CHAPTER EIGHT

Don't Just Stand There . . .

In the blink of an eye, I was living another life. My framed two-lettered college degrees—BA, MA, and JD—had been traded in for another list of two-lettered efforts: PT (physical therapy), OT (occupational therapy), MT (massage therapy), and TC (Tai Chi). I also tried yoga.

More than anything else, I wanted to protect my family and not allow my MS to alter their lives. I wanted to salvage my mental health and stay involved with them at a meaningful level. The disease was in full play, and shooting Avonex® into my thigh every week was the least I could do.

When I finished IV steroids to fight the numbness in my leg, Dr. Thomas suggested that PT would be appropriate. "One of the best things to do after treating an exacerbation with steroids," he said, "is to be evaluated for PT. We want to keep the affected muscles active and slowly restore them. It may not be perfect, but we might be able to get you back to 80 percent of where you were functioning before the numbness."

I agreed, knowing that it was far better than doing nothing. When I mentioned the lingering clumsiness in my hand, Dr. Thomas offered OT as a method of restoring some of the former strength and grip in my hand and fingers. PT would involve working with the leg and foot. Both therapy departments were conveniently located just down the hall from the Neurology Clinic.

Physical, occupational, and other therapies may restore lost functioning, help you learn skills to compensate for disability, and prevent further deterioration.

Both Dr. Thomas and I had the same philosophy about MS: Never concede the loss of any part of the body or mind to multiple sclerosis.

The physical therapist, Jeff, took this credo one step further. "The background notes say that you were a speedskater," he said. "That explains why your legs are in better shape than most of the MS patients that I have seen." When Jeff compared the strength and range of motion of my "MS" leg against my "good" leg, however, it became apparent what I had lost.

"Is it crazy to think that I'll be able to get back on the ice? It's been months since I've been able to hold the edge of the blade on the ice and not hurt myself."

The last time I had been on the ice, I was devastated by the extent of numbness in my calf muscle and foot. When I tried to shift my weight to the affected leg, there was little sensation to hold the transfer. The whole leg wobbled under the pressure to work normally. Quickly shifting back to my other leg, I lightly pushed my way back to the wooden bench and fell down hard onto the seat. As I ripped the clasping tape off the skates, I shed a private tear for my leg. People with walkers or wheelchairs don't have to worry about wearing skates.

"Not only do I think that we can get you back out there," said Jeff, "but maybe you can learn how to stay ahead of MS by strengthening your less-used muscles." It was the same theory as in OT, which utilized a series of elastic resistance bands and finger coordination exercises.

During the second week of PT, the receptionist told me to go directly into the large room of work-out equipment and computer monitors. The room was a cross between a gym, a computer lab, and a four-bed hospital room. I sat down on one of the soft-padded therapy beds and began my limbering-up exercises. Jeff was assisting another physical therapist with a new patient, a man in his mid-50s, who was struggling to walk with an artificial leg.

The man remained perched between parallel bars, clenching the bars with both hands for balance and support. His face was flushed red with effort, and he grunted with discomfort. Jeff walked over to me to make sure that I was comfortable with the warm-up stretches.

"I'll be with you in a minute," he said. "It's his first time on the new leg, and I want to give the other therapist a hand."

My attention was drawn to the man's new prosthetic leg, which was exposed beyond his knee-length hospital shorts. The aches that shot up and down my leg with Jeff's manipulations seemed minor and tolerable by comparison. *Even if my leg is partially numb, at least I still have it to work with,* I thought. Life always has a way of showing me that, whenever I face a new problem, it isn't as bad as I initially feared. Despite the difficulties of overwhelming fatigue, stumbling, and surprising bouts of utterly confounded thinking, I'm still here. Relatively speaking, I had no reason to complain.

In between the pulling and stretching of OT and PT, MT provided the direct benefit of increasing blood circulation without adding physical stress or fatigue. No matter what the initials of these therapies spelled out, they were aimed at fighting MS from all directions.

It's important to stick with a therapy program, but Dr. Thomas and Jeff emphasized that I should avoid pushing myself to exhaustion. They advised me to treat PT and OT like a job commitment, regularly setting aside time to complete the task of improving flexibility, stimulating circulation, and working my muscles to stay ahead of the next MS exacerbation. There were no guarantees, but finally I was doing something constructive to prevent further loss of functioning. But, in addition to my efforts to deal with the physical challenges of MS, I also had to consider the cognitive challenges.

◆ ◆ ◆

"Where are we going!?" I blurted out, pulling the car toward the curb. Meredith and Lauren stopped talking in the backseat. Terri turned and looked at me. We had only driven halfway down our block, and already I couldn't remember why we were in the moving car. I was experiencing a complete *loss of purpose.*

"We're going to visit your grandmother," Terri said calmly. "Remember?"

Of course, she was correct, and we drove on toward the nursing home in silence. I knew exactly where we were going, once I knew what I was doing. I wasn't missing the route—the whole purpose for the travel had disappeared. The sense of being misplaced had a larger meaning beyond searching for a correct address.

Would tying my shoes become a major problem at some point in the future? If I were compelled to concentrate on the twisting and looping process, would I stall before double knotting? Only unconscious, reflexive finger movements were probably saving me from switching to loafers. What other parts of my life will I lose because of the way that MS cuts off chunks of my thinking? Would I even recognize that it was related to MS and that I should do something about it?

I understood numbness in a leg, because I never used to trip or stumble on the stairs.

I knew the blinding fog of optic-neuritis, because I used to enjoy the colors of bright sunny days and well-lit rooms.

I understood slowed cognitive processing, because I used to instantly sort, recall, and articulate on-point information at my litigation fingertips.

I knew delayed recognition, because I could no longer take for granted knowing normally familiar people and objects.

I knew it was MS and that I was disabled by it, because I had witnessed similar disabilities in others.

As sure as all of this was true, I also knew that it wasn't the end of a productive, fulfilling life. I knew that I had been defined by my litigation career, but that was over now, and the rest of my life was just starting. My fight would take place from inside the disease, by acknowledging its changes, and not by slamming headlong against the obstacles presented by MS. Self-taught ways to avoid unnecessary mental jams were not difficult to discover.

> The mental disorientation of MS can be frightening, but it is best to remain calm and safe until it passes. And it probably will pass.

Albert Einstein was once asked for his phone number, but he didn't know it, so he reached for a telephone book to look it up. Obviously,

Mr. Einstein didn't feel compelled to fill his brain with routine details, as long as he knew where to get the information when he needed it. This method of recalling and processing information sounded like the perfect approach for coping with MS cognitive changes. Maintaining a calm openness to let the information flow in at its own pace, and being willing to ask for directions when confused, seemed an amenable path through my stalled mental moments. If the answer isn't at hand right now, give me a moment or two, and I might either remember the information or know where to find it.

I decided to consolidate all of the basic information I needed into one easy, accessible resource to keep track of my life. I acquired a gadget. I had laughed at those electronic handheld devices, and the people who seemed to run their lives by endlessly tapping at a pad. Now, having become a "wall-tapper" because of my need to tap my hands and fingers against walls to maintain my balance and equilibrium, I thought that tapping the palm-size unit was a natural extension, helping me to organize my confusing obligations and information.

At my fingertips were a combined calendar, phone-and-address list, to-do list, and several other programs. It was a great general memory aid. I no longer needed to check three different calendars to determine when I had a doctor's appointment or the number of my uncle's cell phone. It was all in one place, and I took the device with me everywhere.

After a few hours of storing all of my Rolodex and calendared appointments, I was ready. Even the color screen could be adjusted to my hazed vision. In addition, all of the information could be backed up on my home computer with the push of a button.

Electronic handheld devices are very useful for keeping track of appointments and other important information.

"What this?" said Terri, after discovering all of my paper calendars tossed into the garbage.

"I can't continue to rely on a bunch of different lists, calendars, and reminder charts. This single device will keep me going in the right direction. Now, I can avoid that gnawing feeling of always forgetting something."

"Is there anything else that could help?"

"As long as you're asking, please help me keep things where they belong. We don't have to run the house like a hospital, but unless something is being used, then there's no reason why it can't be put back where it belongs. Scissors should be put in the proper drawer after they are used; the same with the Scotch tape or the phone. The kids are definitely the worst culprits. I don't want to yell at the girls about dumb stuff, but the daily searching for things is exhausting." It was simply a matter of needing organization to avoid mental chaos.

"If we have a designated spot for certain items," said Terri, "then it will be easier for the girls to put things away."

"The refrigerator door is another example," I said. "Let's keep notices and invitations on the top door and all of the school artwork and pictures below." Although she may have thought that I was a bit unhinged, Terri agreed to help me stay organized. It was a matter of arranging the important details of our lives so that they would stay front and center in my mind.

"Now you remember that you're picking up the girls after school today," said Terri. "Right?"

Even if I had remembered on my own, I wasn't insulted by the extra prompts. Terri recognized my need for repetition. A tussled sea of scribbled Post-Its™ spread over dresser-tops and tables only confused me further, but now if I couldn't mentally grasp a schedule detail, I could refer to my handheld electronic organizer. Combined with simple techniques of reliable organization to bolster recall, I functioned better with a dependable nexus to basic directions for sorting out the confusing moments. And there were many of them to sort through.

I tried Tai Chi, a form of exercise, but the synchronized movements were impossible to recall. Yoga classes, however, were so calming that some of the students dozed off while lying on the soft-padded floor. The gentle stretching and breathing were as useful as Tai Chi, but without the required group pace and memorization. Both my body and spirit were flexed and tranquil when I left yoga class. It was the still moments of uninterrupted quiet that were useful for mental sorting and physical recharging. These were lessons that I could carry anywhere. Yoga taught me to listen to my body and take better care of myself, reducing the possibility of an MS exacerbation. I responded to all of these different therapies and felt released by becoming more attuned to my body.

All of the therapies for my body were beneficial, but still I wondered if there were activities that would exercise my ability to think. The "use it or lose it" truism also applies to cognitive functioning. Although I wasn't searching for a trendy thinking activity to boost IQ, I was concerned that without use, the speed of my recall and problem solving would continue to diminish. The trick was to find a challenging and rewarding activity that would not add stress.

◆ ◆ ◆

"May I read to your class sometime this week?" I said.

"Are you serious? You'll come and read to my class?" said Terri.

"If they can handle it," I said, smiling at Terri, "then so can I."

I used to speak with the third- and fifth-grade classes on "Career Day," answering questions about how much attorneys get paid. I spoke about helping to correct the injustices in people's lives. and how staying in school was the best way to achieve their dreams. But they usually wanted to know what kind of car I drove and how many secretaries worked for me. It had been difficult to connect with or inspire an entire class within the allotted 20 minutes.

But when I plunked myself down onto a kindergarten-sized chair in Terri's classroom, armed with my Dr. Seuss book and gazing eye-to-eye with a floor full of 5-year-olds, they were with me for every Diffendorfer word. This was not like lecturing to a law-school class. I could reach these children by sharing a great story that made us all smile. After this enjoyable volunteering experience, I received a fat manila envelope in the mail stuffed with notes and colorful drawings of me reading to the class. The children didn't just say "Thanks"; they also pleaded for me to come back and read again.

They will never know it, but I probably gained more from the experience than the students. The value of their innocent appreciation was immeasurable and reminded me of the exhilaration of grassroots volunteering, a feeling that I had not had since working with campers who were disabled. Directly connecting with children was even more satisfying than my former participation as a member of numerous legal committees and nonprofit boards of directors.

Volunteering to help others is often of more value to the volunteer than to the person receiving assistance.

The Milwaukee Public Museum was seeking volunteer docents for a powerful exhibit, "Daniel's Story," which was traveling from the Holocaust Museum in Washington, D.C. The exhibit depicted an epic and tragic account of a Jewish family's demise in Germany during World War II. It was considered a safe introduction for children. In many ways, this was the survival story of my father, his parents, and our extended family in the Warsaw Ghetto.

With a short and well-rehearsed script, along with a stool to rest upon, I would greet school groups for 5–10 hours a week. For several months, I introduced the Holocaust Exhibit to hundreds of schoolchildren and their teachers, often to crowds standing 10 deep and more than 20 across. As I shared "Daniel's Story," and looked into the astonished eyes of the students, I felt that I was keeping alive the memory of my own relatives, as well as the millions of other people who needlessly perished.

Although I was immersed in a valuable mission, there were docent days when my best intentions didn't last very long. Even after just a couple of hours, it was difficult to speak to the eager crowd. On one occasion, when I was unable to finish the question-and-answer period, I passed the podium to another volunteer. Gerald was an 85-year-old Holocaust survivor, and he explained how he miraculously survived the Nazi onslaught. I slumped down onto a folding chair next to him, clenching my hands to avoid a display of shuddering fingers. There was a secluded bench in the Egyptian area near a mummy named DJed-Hor, where I could sit quietly and concentrate on deep breathing—yoga style. Mr. DJed didn't disturb me, and I certainly didn't bother him. After 15 or 20 minutes to recharge my MS-sizzled nerves, my hands were steady enough so that I could refer to my notes without trying to read shaking papers.

MS demanded that I pace myself, whether through a routine matter or the most exhilarating moments. The unwritten goal of volunteering was to be intact at the end of the project and not inflame my MS symptoms. My mind and body were undependable and would rarely function exactly the same way twice. A person facing each day with MS needs to be prepared for varying levels of energy and ability. It's like telling a person that their clothes will fit differently each morning, and, sometimes, their outfits might dramatically change sizes throughout the day.

I had to be prepared to stop and take a break to relax, cool myself down, breathe deeply, and recover some mental focus and physical energy. Remaining unsurprised by fatigue and slowed comprehension was pivotal to riding out the changing landscape of daily life with MS. It was far better to take a necessary mental respite, whether standing in a museum, walking in a park, or driving to visit my grandmother, than to be rattled and forced to walk away from something.

I was unaware that my experiences of MS had been running parallel to the experiences of actor David Landers, otherwise known as *Squiggy* on the '70s television show *Laverne and Shirley*. For many years, Landers had also hidden his MS from friends, family, and career. I met him when he was on a tour promoting his book. Learning how to conceal his numbness and stumbling had merely landed him a reputation as an alcoholic, which had led to unemployment. The 8-foot bookshelves at the Schwartz bookstore, nestled in the Village of Shorewood, provided a sheltered setting for opening the topic of MS and my clandestine disability. Touched by Landers's genuineness and the striking similarity of our guarded symptoms, I felt comfortable sharing a personal coping tip with *Squiggy*, a "trick of the MS trade" that I often used.

"You should lose your socks," I said, pointing at his brown socks. His quirky grin twitched, suggesting that this was not the typical greeting he usually received while on tour. Since Landers had spoken about drudging through similar difficulties with heat and fatigue, I thought that he would appreciate my method for keeping these MS symptoms at bay.

"Do *what* with my socks!?" he said. He seemed to think that I was insulting him, maybe because his socks were brown.

"Lose them," I said. "Don't wear them anymore." My rationale was simple: "Stay as cool as possible at all times without freezing yourself. It's easier to warm up with coffee, if needed, but much more difficult to cool down while holding the heat in." He frowned a bit and began to nod his head.

"I can relate to that!" said Landers. "But why can't I wear my socks?" He raised his eyebrows and looked at his feet.

"You wouldn't wear gloves in a warm room or during the summer, right?" I said. "Then why wear socks that hold in heat and fire up your fatigue?"

He leaned slightly forward and looked down at my sockless ankles. A calm smile stretched across his face, as he perhaps imagined the feel of natural air-conditioning on his feet and lower legs.

"A little odd," said Landers, "but I like that. It's so great when people share the things that help them get through MS."

It began to dawn on me: *Sharing with others might be the best way for me to survive MS.*

My volunteer efforts were strikingly different from my previous organizational involvements. When a volunteering effort arises from an ardent passion to share a topic of personal interest, the experience holds an absolutely crowning sense of fulfillment. Even though I was operating with far lower mental and physical energy limits, it was still better than sitting home and overanalyzing my medical condition. I realized I could still accomplish something of importance despite MS. Plus, it felt good to genuinely connect with other people.

❖ ❖ ❖

There are others out there with MS, and they may be confused, angry, and feeling alone. The newsletter of the Wisconsin Chapter of the National Multiple Sclerosis Society, *MS-Connections*, announced that they were searching for Peer Supporters—people with MS who were willing to talk with folks who have been similarly diagnosed. This sounded like a natural fit, and perhaps it was time for me to help light the path for others with MS.

The thick, red binder lying in front of me on the conference room table held the connections between those people who are already living with MS and those who may not yet know how to survive with MS.

The daylong training for a new group of volunteer Peer Supporters was held at the busy offices of the Wisconsin Chapter of the National Multiple Sclerosis Society. The honeycomb of cubicles and offices buzzed with the mixed energy of scheduling educational programs, the business of fund-raising events, and dissemination of information to callers. The office staff of 25 clearly had their hands full. For me, this energetic crusade meant a whole new world of MS-fighting activity and the realization that I was not alone in dealing with the disease.

Two seasoned staff members led the Information and Referral Division. They walked us through the binder, which listed resources and discussion points for telephone callers. They knew what they were doing and seemed excited about training new telephone volunteers.

"You folks answering calls are often on the front lines," said Diane Baughn, the Information and Referral Director. "Right after people have been diagnosed with MS, they turn to us. It's often one of the most trying times in their lives. What you say to them may be the most informed and reassuring voice that they have heard since leaving the doctor's office with the news."

Although it would take time to absorb the details about making referrals through the MS services network, I felt extremely comfortable listening to callers talk about their diagnosis and how they were coping with exacerbations. If I didn't know how to answer a question, I knew enough to ask someone else in the office for more information.

My first phone call was from a woman who had questions about whether she should tell her boss that she had MS. I did not pretend that I had the only answers for her concerns, but I knew I was uniquely qualified to share my experience. When I offered to send her booklets from the MS Society that discussed disclosure and employment rights, she gladly accepted, and she welcomed a follow-up phone call.

The commitment to being a Peer Supporter for the MS Society was 1 day a week or more if I felt up to the task. Whether I completed the calls at the Peer Supporter desk in the corner of the Chapter's library or took home a small handful of messages, I was rewarded each time that I picked up the phone to speak with someone with MS. By reaching out to inform and connect with callers, I was personally taking a leap forward.

The MS Society, with its nationwide network of chapters, is a supportive resource for people with MS and their families.

Although it was not intended to be a *mask*, the anonymity of sharing through the telephone gave both the caller and me the opportunity to candidly discuss MS without judgment or stigma. It was comfortable for both of us, and I didn't have to act like an attorney to help someone through a turning point. The Peer Supporter role was a valuable experience, but still I wondered, *What else can I do?*

My routine of physical and OT exercises was geared for my particular problem areas and wouldn't necessarily be right for other people with MS. As a volunteer Peer Supporter with the MS Society, I could openly share information and the coping skills I had learned. But, most of all, I listened and didn't assume that "one size fits all." MS is a unique individual experience, and coping with MS is different for each person. I encouraged callers to develop their own distinctive symptom management program in conjunction with their doctors.

The lingering question in being a Peer Supporter was how to address what was described by various callers as "thinking problems." I was quite familiar with the cognitive challenges of MS, but I wondered whether I should discuss the subject with callers, especially when cognitive difficulties were hardly mentioned in the MS brochures. Neurologists were beginning to notice the existence of cognitive problems, but the experiences of actual patients were still noticeably absent from the MS literature.

Studies may have established the existence of cognitive difficulties for MS patients, but it seemed that not all medical professionals fully acknowledged or understood the far-reaching implications. Nothing addressed the underlying problem that MS patients silently face, day in and day out, being unable to articulate their mental disorientation. There was no gathering point of information for MS patients in their shared ordeal of mental challenges.

"My neurologist says that the 'thinking cells' are not affected by my multiple sclerosis," said one caller. *"He said that my trouble*

finding words to finish sentences might be a middle-aged-female thing." Her overall medical picture was unknown to me, and I certainly was in no position to contradict her neurologist, but what she had been told did not sound correct. Glancing through an NMSS brochure, I highlighted references about the existence of cognitive problems in MS patients and mailed it to her, along with a note suggesting that she share the information with her neurologist and perhaps seek another opinion.

I was eager to share my perspective with cognitively challenged callers, but they needed to be guided by more than just my personal coping strategies, especially when they were not being assessed or treated for their cognitive difficulties. Although the questions about cognitive symptoms came from many callers, it wasn't for me to advise them to get a neuropsychological evaluation or to diagnose their problems as being more than just physical.

"*My husband complains that he can't pay attention at work, and that he's forgetting to do things he's agreed to do,*" said one woman. "*Fatigue has been slowing him down, and he's been written up in his personnel record. He's afraid he'll be fired.*"

The MS literature talked about dealing with the emotional side of multiple sclerosis and its relationship to physical fatigue, but this never sounded quite right. I would mail out the brochures dealing with these subjects, but wished that I had more to give.

"*I've been biting off the heads of everyone I work with,*" said an attorney who had been recently diagnosed. "*By the time I get home, I'm yelling at the kids and can't talk to anyone. I don't think it's the MS, because I'm still biking every week and feel great!*" He had no idea how much I could relate to his life. I'd been there and had smacked into those walls.

People who are diagnosed with MS are often immediately concerned with the possibility of disabling physical symptoms. Without warning, however, more than half of them will also be affected by cognitive challenges. For every MS patient who called the MS Society with "thinking" questions, I could only presume that there were many others who remained silent. I was extremely fortunate to be treated by a neuropsychologist and a neurologist who appreciated my cognitive challenges. A large portion of the MS population was possibly like me, ill-prepared to understand and seek treatment for the "thinking" disability of MS. Most people cannot imagine, nor admit to others, that this is indeed happening to them.

Similar to my situation before meeting Dr. Matthais, many callers seemed to be unaware of the hidden cognitive aspects of MS. Through listening to callers and sharing my similar frustrations and coping strategies, I sensed a substantial void in the diagnosis and treatment of this disabling facet of MS. There must be a more direct way to reach out to doctors, patients, and families about the existence of cognitive issues in MS.

◆ ◆ ◆

After retiring from my law practice, I enlisted as an e-mail mentor for Avonex®. If I could mix a medication and inject it into my thigh, then perhaps others could, too. It's natural for a person with MS to question whether they have the fortitude to inject themselves on a regular basis. Doing things that are "good for you" and "necessary" are not automatically acceptable or welcome. After all, this was not a spa treatment.

The purpose of being an Avonex® mentor was not to convince anyone else to take the medication. Rather, it was an opportunity to share my experience of denial, anger, learning, and eventual acceptance of Avonex® as a treatment to fight the progression of MS. Perhaps the confidence that I had gained to face MS with preemptive action might encourage others.

The manufacturers of MS medications have many useful educational resources to offer, including Web sites and support hotlines.

I opened the topic of my MS-related cognitive difficulties in the MS chat room on the Avonex® Web site. I wanted to reach out to others who might have similar cognitive difficulties, so without identifying myself as a Peer Supporter or a mentor, I typed my message:

"Often, I have a 5–15-second delay in recognizing what is going on, what is being said, who I am talking to, or what is supposed to happen next. Don't ask me a compound question unless you want me to shut down completely. One thing

at a time and wait, it will become familiar. Has anyone encountered this difficulty? For those of you who have experienced this type of mental drifting, have you noticed whether or not it seems to get worse over time? I am now 42, and was diagnosed in 1996. Up until about a year ago, I thought MS would just be a physical battle. Thanks for reading and sharing your thoughts, JEFFREY G.

Holding an e-mail breath, I clicked "Enter," and then shut off the computer. They were all out there reading, and within a few days there was a stream of comments by others:

"I have had to deal with exactly what you mentioned. It's like I'm a third person watching myself try to interact with the outside world," said one writer.

"Jeffrey, no, it's definitely not just you. Some words just get harder to find. I try to stay active with crosswords and interesting books," said another person.

"I definitely know your 'slow to respond feeling,'" added one writer. *"Lately, I find myself full of comments and answers, but I'm unable to speak. Sometimes, I have to tell people I'll answer later (after I have a chance to organize my thoughts). Luckily, I no longer work, so my husband understands that sometimes he has to WAIT. I often find myself in a fog and unable to interact with anyone."*

"Hi, Jeffrey," said another. *"Yes! I have experienced this. I let most people think I am just deep in thought, and I avoid long conversations."*

Another gentleman wrote, *"Lately, I've been experiencing some difficulty even thinking of things to say. My wife is starting to feel like I'm pulling away, and I don't want to lose her. It's just that I feel like my head is ... how do I say this? ... feeling cloudy. I was hoping someone out there might know what I'm talking about."*

I certainly did know what they were talking about. Whether they had difficulties remembering passwords at work, detailed instructions, finding words, or being able to state their address, it was a pervasive problem in the MS community. This was well beyond frustration and disability. The disruption was devastating, reaching into their lives and homes, silently halting daily functioning. As I quietly read the familiar, yet unseen agony of these MS patients, I knew that there were thousands more who would never read the chat-room discussion. They may feel alone in coping with their mental disconnections, but there is something positive that they can do. It will never happen, however, unless patients and their doctors understand the impact of MS on cognitive abilities.

The monthly publication of the NMSS, *InsideMS,* opened the discussion of emotional and cognitive aspects of MS, acknowledging that everything from depression to forgetfulness was part and parcel of the MS package. Editorial letters confirmed that readers were privately knocked back on their heels by cognitive disruptions and were disturbed by their doctors' lack of knowledge.

How can people with MS feel comfortable sharing their cognitive challenges with their doctors if medical professionals do not understand or fully appreciate the problem? Patients are left to believe that it must be "something else" that is making them lose their minds, so they keep their cognitive difficulties to themselves. Clearly, there needs to be a far broader discussion about MS patients who live with the cognitive distortions of the disease.

There needs to be a broader discussion of the cognitive challenges of MS.

◆ ◆ ◆

"You should write a book about your cognitive challenges," said Dr. Matthais.

"I can barely focus on reading a newspaper," I said, "so how can I write a book? Who would read it?"

"I think you would find a lot of people out there with MS who could really relate to your experiences, and who would benefit from your perspective. It's not any different than what you are already doing through the MS Society, except that you would be able to reach more people—sooner than one phone call at a time. I'm also sure that doctors would benefit from your insight."

I concluded that she was probably right. There were no other books available that presented life from inside the mental twister of MS. However, trying to write one myself might take a very long time, given my strained focus. Some people have said that when they chronicled their personal journey through a major illness, it served as a release for their emotions, as well as helped them stay mentally sharp. Brain flexing couldn't hurt me, but I questioned whether I was the right person to bring up the subject. Should I bare my soul when there were other ways (such as being a Peer Supporter and an Avonex® mentor) to *anonymously* address concerns and questions from other people with MS?

The answer to the challenge presented by Dr. Matthais was immediately obvious: Reach out as wide as possible to the MS population and its supporting networks. It is best to talk openly to someone about MS, whether on the telephone, face-to-face, or in a memoir written for other patients.

"I'll start making diary-type notes about what has been going on and see if it makes any sense," I told Dr. Matthais.

"I think it will be good for you to write about your experiences," she said, "and how you have worked through the various issues. It would be especially useful for others involved with MS to read about it."

Tips for Living
It's More Than Just Sitting Through a Series of Appointments

- ◆ Ask your doctor what you can do to remain mentally and physically healthy, beyond taking medication.
- ◆ If your concerns seem ignored, or you are repeatedly left with unclear answers, then get a second qualified medical opinion. You should have the doctor's total attention when you are in the examining room.
- ◆ Never give in to MS. Multiple sclerosis exacerbations do not have the final word. Ask your neurologist for a referral to

occupational, physical, or massage therapy, or any other kind of mind or body therapy that might prevent deconditioning and teach you strategies for the improvement of thinking and movement.

Taking a Different Path

◆ Retiring from a career is choosing to do something different that is challenging and interesting—but not detrimental to your overall health.

◆ Give up thinking there are "no options" in your current situation and realize there is a wide-open arena of choices.

◆ You will find time and quiet opportunities for contemplation in retirement, but make a promise to yourself to keep your mind active. Whether it is reading books, doing crossword puzzles, keeping a diary, or writing an editorial letter, do something to challenge your mind. Maintain your cognitive functions by actively using them—or risk losing them.

◆ Maintaining clear thinking spaces in your life means saying "no" to some requests. A trusted family member or friend can be a practical filtering device to sift through incoming requests for your limited energy.

◆ Ask for clarification, reminders, and direction when a situation is confusing.

◆ When faced with a moment of befuddlement, don't force it. Give yourself permission to pause and breathe calmly; relax and patiently gather your thinking focus. Allow yourself the time and mental space to ride out your *temporary* lapses in thinking.

◆ Limit visual distractions and live an uncluttered life. Clear floors and tabletops; organize shelves and drawers. Hold an annual rummage sale and sell unused items that you won't miss anyway.

◆ Keep lists for daily responsibilities and activities, displaying them in a handy manner for quick additions and deletions. Also keep a list of short-term and long-term projects, remembering there is a difference between the effort and time required for each set of goals.

Each Day

◆   Prioritize your activities.

◆   Have a sense of purpose and accomplish something.

◆   Renew and maintain bonds with family and friends.

◆   Establish a minimum exercise routine and do it religiously.

◆   Find ways to relax and soothe your mind to prevent or ease stress.

◆   Seek a spiritual connection within your church or synagogue and with the nature that surrounds you.

◆   Find pleasure and peace within yourself and surroundings— perhaps through music, nature walks, the scent of a burning candle, or talking with a friend or family member.

◆   Remember to have fun, and make it a part of your regular schedule. Permit yourself to laugh out loud, especially at yourself. Watch funny movies and attend comedy shows and plays.

◆   Be patient with yourself by taking breaks and extra time to complete projects, spreading them out over several days, if necessary.

CHAPTER NINE

Taking the Middle Fork

My legs were still twitching on the way home, after the stretching workout of physical therapy. I've always preferred driving the lakeside route along Milwaukee's Lake Michigan shoreline. The left view offered hills and tree-covered bluffs, topped by ornate condo towers. The lake rhythmically washed up onto Bradford Beach on my right. This was the best place to watch the sunrise, Independence Day fireworks, the start of the circus parade, and Saturday morning fundraising walks. The route had texture.

Cruising at 35 miles per hour was the perfect speed to blow through the three stop lights that controlled the 7-mile stretch. It never made much sense to speed up only to wait at a red light. The bulk of the city traffic drove on top of the bluff, stopping for buses, cabs, and orange construction cones. Down here along the water there were waves of calm. During the day or night, snow or rain, I knew the lake route as confidently as bats maneuvering catacombs in the dark. The road stretched out like a private driveway to my home.

It was a sunny day in late March, and I relaxed as I listened to the rhythmic pounding of the alternative rock station. Anticipating the turn up the Lafayette Hill toward my house, I stayed in the left lane for several miles after exiting the freeway ramp. I followed the taillights of a blue Toyota into the left turn lane, and then both of us stopped at the red light.

Suddenly, the boat slips on my right and the tennis courts on my left were all wrong. The brake lights in front of me went off as the driver turned left. *If this isn't the right direction*, I wondered, *should I still follow the Toyota, and hope that I don't pull up in front of the driver's house instead of mine?*

This is not right. I missed the turn! Of course, it had to be the correct turn, but the landmarks were new—familiar but changed in a way so that even the shapes were less defined. *Pull forward again. There are only two more oncoming cars before I can turn.* How could I suddenly be so far off the mark, overshooting my turn to the point that I didn't know where I was in the city? The Toyota's lights had turned and were halfway up the hill, leaving me alone in the crossroad and stalled by overwhelming hesitation. With no opposition, the approaching cars quickly cleared the junction, but I vacillated, not wanting to turn onto an unfamiliar street. Someone behind me honked, demanding I go through the open intersection. *But where was I going?*

The mental disorientation of MS can be frightening, but it is best to remain calm until it passes.

The horn blasted again, louder this time, as I lifted my hands in exasperation, not wanting to be forced into a driving error. Executing the unidentified turn onto an unfamiliar street filled me with the same trepidation as accelerating to drive off a cliff. *This must be payback for all of my prior driving impatience.* A quick glance in the rearview mirror confirmed that the car behind me was pressed at my tail and preparing to drive through my trunk. But the horn still did not convince me that the turn would lead to my house, so I pulled out, swerving back into the driving lane. I began following a Volvo through the intersection. *Now what?* I wondered.

Maybe I should turn around. Maybe I should call Terri. Trying to verbalize my bafflement left me even more confused, and I decided that calling her from behind the wheel might be more distracting than productive. Besides, why put Terri on the phone just so she can listen to me swear in frustration? This was no time for cell phones.

Stick with the Volvo. The commercials say it is a very safe car, although that may not help me if I'm just following one around the city. I started repeating aloud: *Don't leave the lane; follow the taillights,* as if I needed to convince myself that this was the best way to stay focused. I continued to drive, but it was difficult to understand or anticipate exactly what should happen next. I lost the ability to do anything other than watch for the Volvo's brake lights.

I passed an empty beach on my right, but it did nothing for my recollection—it had nothing to do with me. Where are the familiar road signs and landmarks? There were none on this stretch of road, and the trees were just trees. As the road curved, I felt pulled by a vacuum of nonexistence into a place where I did not belong and could not escape. It didn't matter that I was just going home.

My confusion was stunning as I pondered my location. Was my driving erratic? Although the sound of horns had ceased at the intersection, and cars were not swerving to avoid me, my driving might be unreliable. I just wasn't sure. Before unwittingly driving off the road, I decided to pull over and stop in the empty right-hand parking lane. I put the car in "park," slowly closed my eyes, and turned on the air conditioning.

This is ridiculous, I thought. I opened my eyes and observed that the steering wheel was exactly where I had left it, arched toward the curb. Someone had switched the road on me, like a clever *Candid Camera* stunt. I knew the date and my name. I knew my car and what I had done earlier that day. Idling at a complete stop, the car stereo gently carried a Sarah McLachlan song saying something about "pulled from the wreckage" and being "in the arms of the angel." The words echoed through my head as I contemplated the overtone of her message.

My hands released the wheel and slid down into my lap, as if acknowledging that the car could do nothing without me. The release of the seatbelt allowed my body to shift sideways in the driver's seat so I could look out of the passenger's side window. My vision was drawn out of the car by the brightened, yet soft colors of the grass, trees, and water. It seemed as if their edges were trying to blend together. I had driven into a French Impressionist painting *somewhere* near my house.

Maybe it was just the MS fog that obstructed my left eye, only now it was messing with both eyes. For several years, there had been a permanent blockage in my left field of sight. Perhaps it had now been amplified by driving in direct sunlight. MS had challenged the crisp clarity of my sight, but it had never altered my recollection of what I was seeing or where I was, so I ruled out this possibility.

Maybe this was similar to the whole psychedelic drug thing of the '60s, but I hadn't wanted to hallucinate then, and certainly not now. If I was about to lose consciousness, then at least I was parked, but if this was a hallucination, then parking the car wouldn't necessarily stop it from floating away. This was a very disappointing and rather unimaginative fantasy without any flying monkeys and talking trees. There was no dream to come out of. It was just me, the car, and some blurred, rearranged pieces of my daily puzzle.

> The mental lapses of MS are unpredictable and can occur without any obvious catalyst. Memories are not erased but can be more difficult to access.

I felt no clear emotion at the moment, and it didn't occur to me that I might be justified in simply freaking out on the spot and pounding on the windows. The events of the day had been unremarkable, nothing new there. There was no inner avoidance mechanism inducing me to stay away from home. The only danger would be to emotionally overstate the significance of the moment and work myself into a frenzy. Whatever was happening would be explained at some point, but probably not now, not here on the side of the road.

Similar to other prior MS exacerbations, this mental trip was probably temporary, and my best action was to just sit back, let it pass, and listen to the music. This was easy to do, and a far better alternative than allowing myself to be rattled and overcome by the event. I reminded myself to *stay cool.*

This decision permitted me to feel in control, letting the moment flow toward me head-on, instead of struggling to elude it. Being in control doesn't always mean fighting. The worst thing I could do would be to waste energy by fueling fear and panic. Those reserves were needed to steer safely through what must be another *loss of presence.* I realized that my hands had grasped the steering wheel again. The color returned to my white knuckles as I released my clenched grip. The car would not disappear if I let go. *Relax and let this pass.*

I cranked up all four notches on the air-conditioning unit and turned the cool air vent toward my face, plunging the interior of the car back into the Ice Age. Freezing out a potential MS exacerbation usually helped—although this current experience might not be about heat. My left wrist gently rested against the frigid window vent, chilling the blood flow.

Something would happen to put the road back the way I remembered it. Shifting my gaze to the dashboard, I again confirmed that this was my car. I still knew my name, the amount of our real estate taxes, and that Bill Clinton was President, but now I had a deeper understanding of Dorothy in the Land of Oz, who also just wanted to go home. The highway that had deposited me here was somewhere else, and the averted turn up the hill was behind me without an accessible U-turn in sight. I looked out through the windshield at the road ahead. It bent out of sight, but at some point it *must* offer another route to double back home. Even though only a minute had passed since the missed turn, it seemed like an hour. The logic of remaining parked here indefinitely was fading, along with my patience.

What is all this? I said loudly, to no one in particular. My whole world had become unrecognizable, and I demanded an explanation where there was none. Fear never had a chance to "get in the car," because all I could feel was fury. *I'm doing this to myself*, I yelled at the steering wheel. There was no *figuring out* what to do about it, because I had no idea what *it* was. This stupid disease couldn't tell the difference between deadening a limb and blocking a simple memory!

Making an abrupt decision, fueled by frustration, my foot hit the gas pedal hard enough to press me back into the seat as I pulled the car out of the parking lane and into traffic—going somewhere forward. The road curved right and then left to a red light. Suddenly, the fog lifted! *This is the Lake Drive intersection! I know the house on the corner, the Alumni mansion over my shoulder, and the next street should be ... Marietta, three blocks from my house.* Everything was as perfectly clear as it had always been—except for what had just happened. After steering left and driving a few blocks, I pulled in behind Terri's car, which was parked in front of our house. The mail was waiting, as usual, sticking out of the overstuffed mailbox.

The clock on the dashboard showed that the entire event had occurred in less than a few minutes! Yet, to me, it had crawled by like an entire day, stretching time into eternity.

Was it amnesia and hallucination at the same time? I was thankful that the experience had not involved hearing voices or seeing dogs carrying computers, although it had been an entangling effort to just do nothing, feeling helpless while hoping that I was harmless to others. Staying calm, while cautiously moving forward, had helped me get through it.

Having no clear grasp of the mental quicksand that I had just driven through, I cringed at the thought of telling Terri, but she listened carefully and stared past me, seemingly taken aback by the frightful image of my losing recognition while driving. The inevitable question quickly followed.

"Do you feel safe to drive again?" There was the rub. How could I answer her when I didn't know if this was going to be an isolated incident? How could anyone believe that it was safe for me to drive when I had lost my bearings just a couple of miles from home on a route that I had driven thousands of times? Nightmares pass after waking up, but I hadn't been asleep. I took solace in the fact that I still knew how to operate a car and that I had not gone through a red light or caused an accident.

"Driving wasn't the problem," I said, "but *where* I was driving was the sticking point. I can't wait to tell Dr. Matthais about this. There must already be a thick 'Going Nuts' section in my file at the hospital. They'll need a second folder just for the next appointment."

"Do you think it's the MS?" said Terri.

"It better be, because I'm not up for a new disease to deal with."

"Is this the first time something like this has happened?" said Terri.

"Like this, yes. There was nowhere to go to get away from it—and then it was over."

It felt as though I had been losing small pieces of myself. When MS stopped me on the side of the road, I was forced to look around and see that chunks were indeed missing. Earlier in the week, I had caught myself suddenly aware of having gone outside and unsure of why I was there and why I had left the house.

"Are you going up or down?" said Terri. She waited for me to make a move on the stairs, a place that had stopped me before.

"Haven't decided yet," I said. Then I smiled and decided to go up for no particular reason.

During the past few months, I had frequently become so immersed in clogged conversations that I relied more and more on Terri to relate the discussion to me, sometimes slowly. Working together saved us from losing or tripping over each other. Chuckling and shaking my head at my own silence, people assumed that I had been contemplating their last comment, but the truth was that I had lost their words and only heard the mumbled sounds of their speech.

When I shared my driving confusion with Drs. Matthais and Thomas, neither of them reacted with any clinical surprise. They consulted privately with each other and came up with two possible theories. Although it had not been a physical manifestation, such as numbness in my hand, face, or leg, MS was the obvious answer. They decided on testing to make sure that MS was indeed the culprit.

"Have you ever had an EEG?" said Dr. Thomas. This sounded electrical, and I silently prayed that shock therapy had been outlawed in Wisconsin.

"No, I haven't, but I have a feeling you're about to recommend it." It was becoming difficult to hold my cooperative smile in place. Suddenly, having a few lingering numb fingers and toes didn't seem so bad.

"There is a small, but unlikely chance that you are experiencing a type of brain seizure, which may be causing these lapses," he said. "An EEG will help us rule it out."

The EEG is a test that records brain function. It may be used to rule out the possibility of mini-seizures.

The possibility of mini-seizures was too serious to ignore; though I agreed to the testing, I did not want to stay overnight in the hospital during the required 24-hour computer hook-up monitoring. Being wired to a small monitor on my belt during the day seemed easy enough to conceal from our daughters, and being attached to the larger computer box would only be necessary while sleeping at night. It was just a couple of wires. No problem, right?

"How many more of these electrodes do you have to attach?" I asked the clinic technician, as the "eleventeenth" wire was being cemented to my scalp and hair roots.

"Just a few more," he said, lying to the back of my head by not offering even a vaguely close number. My question probably made him forget the number, forcing him to start the wiring procedure over without counting the ones already in place. "I'm sorry about the cement fumes," he said. "If winter hadn't returned today, I would open the windows for some air circulation."

The toxic combination of cement fumes and hair tugging closed my eyes. I lost count after 15, or was it 150?

"It's best to leave your arms down and crossed in your lap to avoid snagging a stray wire," he said. The wires gently tapped against the side of my head and flowed down over my shoulders, resembling Jamaican braids. Would it have been easier to hide the EEG if I had agreed to the hospital stay? Once I was at home, how could I avoid Meredith, who insists that my lap is the only location for her late afternoon nap? Were the children ready to confront MS? If not, were these wires and binding the correct introduction? Finally, I decided: *Tell nothing to the kids. Don't let them see me like this.*

I lost count of the number of electrodes. *Multiple sclerosis? What's that?* It felt like he had wound about 3–4,000 yards of gauze around my head to hold the contacts and wires in place. When he was finished, I slowly stood up, as if posturing to balance textbooks on my head. Then I looked at my reflection in the mirror. "So this is what treating major head trauma looks like," I said, examining the white, football helmet-sized binding. He didn't smile. For him, this was a serious procedure.

"Does your coat have a large hood?" he said.

"No, a small one, but if you help me pull it up, it will probably cover the back of my head." I pulled my hat down over the coiled binding, covering the white gauze, and the technician slid the hood up. Perspiration broke out along my hairline. It was still only March, but overheating, weakness, and imbalance seemed only minutes away. Finally, wires and computer attached, I was free to leave.

"Enjoy your day," said the receptionist, glancing up from her computer screen. *She must be kidding*, I thought to myself. Neither her farewell nor my silent smile were genuine.

Wearing a hat pulled down to my eyebrows was normal, given the wind chill. I struggled to keep the hood up over the swollen hat, in an attempt to conceal the gauze protruding down the back of my neck. As I tucked the arms of my sunglasses through the tautly wound material, I reflected on television sketches of the Unibomber.

For years, I had fought to keep MS out of the house to protect our young daughters, but there was no camouflaging this crown of gauze. As I carried the attached computer mainframe through the front door, I braced myself for their possible questions and loss of childhood innocence. Fortunately, they were not home.

> Honest communication is the best way to get through difficult MS cognitive situations. Avoid misunderstandings with others through an informed discussion of those moments.

Later, from my bedroom upstairs, I could hear the clinking of silverware as they finished dinner without me. "Daddy was very tired," Terri explained, "so he went to sleep before we came home." At 8 o'clock, the sound of quick-pounding footsteps up the stairs signaled their bedtime.

"How do you want to handle this?" Terri said. She sat in the dark on the edge of our bed. "Do you want to skip the good-night kiss?"

"No, but be careful that they don't move the covers from around the equipment or my head." Terri returned to the bathroom to help the girls get ready for bed. Through the closed door, I could hear them rinsing their Cinderella toothbrushes and the toothpaste cap falling into the sink.

A struggle began to scratch an itch on my encased scalp. Would the coat-hanger trick work as it once had years ago with a cast on my arm? The heat generated under the comforter began to build. A ski hat was stretched over the binding, and my head felt like it was trapped in a firing kiln. It was too tight for entry under or escape from the wrapping. The heat-itch spread under my pressed hair until it became one massive twitch that screamed to be scratched.

"Maybe I'll tell them you're already asleep, and you'll see them in the morning," said Terri through the cracked door.

"But I'm going to look like this in the morning," I said. "They'll be worried if they don't see me until after school tomorrow. Let's deal with this now, but keep the lights off."

"I'm still glad you didn't check into the hospital," said Terri.

She was right. We would get past this, too. Being at home with MS was far better than being anywhere else with MS. The truth was that, although I didn't really know what Terri thought about seeing me being injected with medications, attached to wires, and becoming a regular hospital visitor, she was always by my side. Without any words, her hand resting on my arm said it all.

After Terri had carefully rearranged the blankets and pillows to conceal my gigantic, gauze-wrapped skull, I was ready for the girls. Under the cloaked darkness of the room, she quickly shuttled Lauren and Meredith past me on their way to bed.

"Are you playing hide-and-seek?" said Lauren, stopping to peer into the blankets in an attempt to see my face.

"You found me! Daddy is in bed before you!" Good-night kisses would be in the dark, and so was I, listening through the door about the Three Billy-Goats Gruff and the menacing Troll living under the bridge.

> Laughter brings people together and is a survival path through MS. Use it often.

◆ ◆ ◆

"It's very similar to the courtroom incident," said Dr. Matthais, "when your client and case notes didn't look familiar."

"But I wasn't stressed out by driving home. It's the same route every day."

"There is no correlation between the appearance of brain lesions on an MRI and what you might be feeling at the moment of the test. In the same way, you can have moments of mental confusion without something specific setting them off."

This was a good description of the times when I felt my mental clarity slipping away. There was no warning when I lost a train of thought; no triggering incident or racing heart to give notice. Everything was just gone—vaporized without a trace—until things returned to normal.

During the MS disconnections, my brain was forced to find different paths to continue the flow of a thought, or, in this case, to remember what was normally familiar. My brain might be able to rewire a new pathway, but the route might take longer. This additional recognition time left me blank.

"How far will this go?" I said. "I guess the short delays are not so bad, as long as I know it's temporary."

"Research suggests that there is no permanent memory loss in MS, but the speed of information recovery can vary depending on the individual," said Dr. Matthais.

Research suggests that there is no permanent memory loss in MS, although brain lesions sometimes cause a slowdown of mental processing, delaying retrieval of information.

The EEG testing had two immediate results: It eliminated the possibility that seizures were causing my recognition lapses (for which I was quite grateful), and it greatly increased my religiosity. Undergoing an EEG wouldn't kill me, nor would dozens of MRIs. Cumulative hours of lying in an MRI chamber and being head-wrapped for an EEG gave me pause to take stock of my health and where it was headed. It was enough to make me stop at my synagogue more often. My physical therapist didn't list sitting down to pray as part of my exercise regimen, but it felt just as useful. Echoing the challenges of physical disability, cognitive numbing was also classic MS. It transcended standard assumptions of what an MS disability should look like by imperceptibly short-circuiting the mind, while visibly crippling the body.

The *extra fork* in the road that I had unexpectedly encountered was, in fact, the same as the smaller incidents that had been occurring for quite some time, only much larger. Apparently, the cognitive confusion of my MS was not limited to stressful moments—the scarred and severed nerve connections in my brain could cause a problem at any time, even during moments of routine and relative tranquility.

Tips for Living

- Stop and pause, if necessary, especially if safety is a concern. Pull yourself away from any situation that confuses you. Give yourself a few quiet moments in an isolated place to allow the world to come back into focus. Loss of recognition is temporary—wait it out calmly.
- Provide yourself with communication back-up, such as a cell phone with a few key preprogrammed numbers for easy reference. This type of security, even if you never use it, can be reassuring.
- Keep a record of delayed recall moments and show it to your neurologist, ensuring that your cognitive challenges receive the appropriate monitoring and treatment.
- Prepare your family and friends by telling them about your moments of disorientation.
- Communication with a spouse, a significant other, or an understanding caregiver is crucial, because they can help you get through the disorienting moments.
- Sharing your difficulties honestly will help you maintain closeness with others.
- Give yourself extra time to learn new information or to recall previously known information.

CHAPTER TEN

Drifting and Dragging in a Mental Wheelchair

A woman was sitting a couple of seats away from me. She seemed preoccupied and continued to look off in the distance without taking notice of me. Lingering in my seat, I stared at her without her noticing. At least, I didn't think she was paying any attention to me. I didn't want her to see me staring, but I was inside, and suddenly flipping on sunglasses to hide my eyes would look ridiculous and draw her attention.

Her face was unfamiliar, and I felt confused by it. Slightly younger than me, nearing 40, she seemed to be completely at ease. Wrapped in a cable-knit wool sweater, she was comfortably fixated on an object off in the distance, unaware that I had been drawn in by her face. My eyes followed the firm curve of her smooth cheekbones and bright gentleness of her eyes. I was torn between the comfort I felt sitting near her and the awkwardness of staring, hoping to avoid her detection. Quickly standing up and walking away would expose that I had no original purpose for sitting there in the first place. Yet, how could I walk away? Deep inside, I somehow knew that she was Terri, my wife.

People have dreams like this. I knew where I was, and who I was looking at, but in some indescribable way everything looked different. The only difference was that in a dream it wouldn't be bothersome. Black and white Rod Serling didn't walk into our living room and introduce the scene as one of his "studies." There was no waking up. Having misplaced my wife on our couch, I was caught frozen by another startling recognition blur in the most taken-for-granted setting: my own home.

We were watching a new episode of *The West Wing*, and Terri didn't notice my bewilderment as I sat quietly near her. Tonight's episode revealed that the show's main character, President Bartlett, was dealing with his startling public disclosure of his MS. I ignored the irony that I was using a TV story about an MS cover-up as a diversion to conceal one of my own mental episodes. MS can be a rather amusing disease in this way, except that Bartlett was only the *pretend* leader of the free world—and had a script that occasionally included MS—whereas I had a young family, and my episodes of MS were real.

The mental lapses of MS are unpredictable and can occur without any obvious catalyst.

For no particular reason, I noticed the length of Terri's hair, which she had intentionally grown past her shoulders over the winter months. Although surprised to realize the length, I was not dumbfounded by the natural process of its growth and direction.

Questions began to arise: Why am I confused now, why here? And most importantly: When would my memory click back in? Maybe I could safely force it by employing routine. "I'm going to make some coffee," I said. "Would you like some?"

"Sure, if you're making it," Terri said. It was my living room, couch, TV, and coffeemaker. It should have been just as obvious that she was Terri, my wife, but it wasn't. The mask was "back on" in the house, but this time, there would be no hiding from myself.

◆   ◆   ◆

"I knew that she was my wife," I told Dr. Matthais, at my next appointment. "It just didn't look like her! I kept staring at her facial features, and it was like I was noticing her appearance for the first time. Her face wasn't the same, not as I recalled it."

It was like watching an old family movie, but one of the characters had been switched. Having known Terri for almost 20 years, the sudden shift was not exactly a romantic notion.

"So what did you do? How long did it last?"

"It was 9:00 P.M., but it seemed like a good time to get up and make coffee, before she noticed anything. I thought my mind would quickly return to normal, like during the driving incident, but staring at her did not trigger anything." As I described for the first time the image-struck evening, it shocked me. The words echoed in my head as if spoken by someone else—someone who had lost his mind. The image of the event stunned me and hung in the room, unclaimed by anyone.

Dr. Matthais was silent, and slightly nodded her head.

MS had slowed me down, but was it now pulling me into dementia? Terri had walked into the living room and sat down, but when I walked in, someone else was sitting in her place. It was haunting. Getting a little lost while driving home was one thing, but this was over the top on the "marital-sanity scale."

I was frustrated and angry. There are certain things in life that I feel entitled to take for granted. Instant recognition of the people I love is one of them. There should be no hesitation or second guessing. No need for a 15-second visual lead-in before engaging in conversation. *She's my wife; it's Terri!*

"I've read all of the MS Society publications," I said, "and there was no mention of anything like this!"

We have been receiving the MS mailings for the past several years, but even though the mailing labels were addressed to me, many of the articles were not. The published emphasis tended to explore the complicated and progressive aspects of physical disability. I needed this information, but where were the instructive articles acknowledging cognitive difficulties?

As I related the story about the ordeal in my living room, Dr. Matthais listened closely. She continued to nod her head in understanding, but her face tightened with concern. *Did she think I was crazy? Maybe I should just shut up before she keeps me in the hospital for observation.*

"Were you able to talk to Terri about what you were experiencing when you looked at her?" she said.

"Hell, no! Why scare her? How can I tell her that her husband doesn't recognize her?" It seemed selfish and cruel. It didn't happen every day, but the momentary delay of recognition had been occurring on a more frequent basis, when I least expected it. "It happens during routine moments and lasts maybe fifteen seconds," I said.

"Can you give me some examples?" While Dr. Matthais waited for an answer, I silently reviewed recent events:

Earlier that week, I had suddenly stopped while walking up the kitchen stairs, unsure of where I was or where I was headed. This wasn't the first time I had gotten lost in my house, so I continued up the stairs, hoping the reason would come back to me. I reached the second floor and, after pausing for a few seconds, I went back down the stairs, still confused.

Two days later, I slid into the front seat of my car and sat in utter amusement looking at the "new" radio and temperature dashboard panel, while also knowing that it was the same as the night before. Slightly shaking my head in disbelief, I ignored it and started the car. Different stairs, car, or road—perhaps it didn't really matter. Shake it off and keep moving! But, the couch ordeal seemed very different. It went beyond all of the prior quirky episodes.

> MS cognitive challenges that remain hidden will continue to cause suffering. Strategies for successfully coping with those difficulties may be found through open discussion.

"When Terri joined me later in the kitchen for coffee, everything was fine. It's impossible to discuss it while it's happening, and it seems absurd to talk about it when it is over."

"If you were in a troubled marriage, there would be other, more obvious answers for this. But from all I've learned about your family life, it's stable and secure."

This one point I was happy to agree with, especially since it hadn't even occurred to me as a possible cause. Suddenly, I was filled with the significance of the next benchmark question.

"Has this incident happened more than once? Not recognizing a familiar face?" said Dr. Matthais.

I paused and stared at her diplomas on the wall, not wanting to hear the answer from my own mouth. Dr. Matthais was waiting for an answer, and there was no turning back. The thought of slipping into denial, escorted by apparent memory deterioration, seemed more dangerous than staying out in the open and waiting for answers. There were never answers in the denial closet, only the darkness of delay.

"Not as dramatic, but more times than I want to recall," I said. There, the door had been kicked wide open, but there was *no* look of surprise on Dr. Matthais's face. It seemed as if she had anticipated my response.

The cognitive challenges of MS can include not immediately recognizing familiar faces and places.

"Can you imagine the predicament," I continued, "of approaching the usual morning good-bye kiss, and becoming suddenly uncertain of who is on the other end of it—with kids standing next to me waiting to be taken to school? I know she is Terri, but I've caught myself hesitating, waiting for the casual recognition. I tell myself to stop questioning the obvious and move on. I've learned to not challenge the lapses. They vanish as soon as we are out the door."

"Does it happen more often during the morning or evening?" said Dr. Matthais.

"There's no reliable pattern, if that's what you mean. I can *lose* her at the most uncommon moments, as well as during the routine encounters of a married couple with two young children and a cat. So what's that?" I was becoming impatient. The more I described the lack of recognition, the more I became disappointed in my ability to cope with the disorientation.

"Has she picked up on your hesitation?" said Dr. Matthais.

"I don't think so, because when the pause is obvious, I smile, look at her, and say right in the middle of the embrace or kiss, 'Wife, right?' She smiles, and seems to think nothing of the comment, probably because I don't act concerned. Fortunately, she agrees with me every time. But it makes me feel uncomfortable and a little sad."

"What about the children?"

"Them, too! Sometimes when I bend down to give one of our girls a kiss on the forehead, I think … Wait! … Do I know her? … Do I have the right child? … Check first! All of the second guessing happens in a few seconds. Fortunately, there is always something that tells me to go ahead and finish what I started. I become more of a bystander at that point, not wanting to do or say anything. Then, before I know it, everyone has gone out the door to school, and I'm back sitting at the kitchen table trying to replay what just occurred. Between the drifting focus of figuring out where I am and who is with me, and my body limping and dragging from numbness and fatigue, MS really sucks!"

"Why haven't you told Terri about this?" said Dr. Matthais.

"It will scare her, won't it? If she is always wondering whether I recognize her or not, won't it push her away?"

"Just think for a minute about how you would feel if this was happening to her instead of you. Wouldn't you want to know about it so you could be supportive and work through it together? Would you want her to keep it to herself and deal with it alone?"

The barrage of direct questions exposed a double standard in my thinking. Protecting myself from openly dealing with these delays was not protecting Terri from anything. If the situation was reversed, I would insist on knowing what was happening. To pretend that I solely owned the problem would have been the worst thing, the most selfish thing that I could have done.

"You're absolutely right," I said, "so *you* tell her!"

"That's not quite the same." Dr. Matthais smiled at the suggestion.

"You know you are not alone with this type of MS problem," she continued. "I recently had another MS patient describe a similar experience. One morning she looked into the bathroom mirror and didn't recognize her own face. Somehow it was different, not the same face that she usually saw looking back at her. It took her a couple of days before she recognized herself."

I wanted to ask whether the woman preferred the new face or her original face, but I knew the answer would always be the comfort of familiarity. At least, for me, it would be.

"The delay in recognition is also your brain's way of trying to find another path around the one that has been cut off by the MS lesions eating through the myelin coating around the nerves. Sometimes, the brain will try to rewire itself around the damaged connections where the myelin coating is gone. Recognition may be slower or may not work at all, causing you to experience delay in processing thoughts," said Dr. Matthais.

"How bad can this get?" I said.

"It's difficult to say whether it will get any worse. About half of MS patients have cognitive difficulties similar to the slowed mental processing that you experience, but only 10 to 15 percent of them have severe cognitive impairment, and you are not there. Taking medication, retiring from work, reducing stress, talking to Terri, and coming to see me—these are all the right things to minimize your cognitive challenges. You're in a better position to deal with this than many other MS patients, especially those who do not even know what is happening to them."

I appreciated her positive attitude. We returned to the subject of telling Terri. "The decision is yours, but are you ready to tell your wife about all of this?" said Dr. Matthais.

"You weren't going to let me out of here without making a decision, were you? I guess the trick is to pick a time when the kids are out of earshot," I said.

Dr. Matthais was right. Why wait to share my experience with Terri, when MS was hitting this hard at home? If widespread cognitive delay could cut off my thinking at random, I questioned whether *everyone* I knew was a potential candidate for my memory disruption. Fortunately, I had learned from my prior experiences with recognition delays not to panic. Just relax, put myself in a safe situation, and let it pass. Any delays with recalling people, even family members, might clear up the same way.

Honest communication is the best way to get through difficult situations.

❖ ❖ ❖

"Remember last week, when I had an appointment with Dr. Matthais?"

Terri looked at me but said nothing as she carried her empty plate to the counter. "There was a special reason for that appointment." I usually clean up the dishes, but I remained seated as Terri started loading the glasses into the dishwasher. She glanced up, indicating that I should continue. "Something MS-bizarre happened, and this time it included you," I said

"What did I do?" she said.

"Nothing, nothing at all," I quickly answered, "and you wouldn't necessarily have ever noticed anything." She joined me at the kitchen table. As I glanced out of the window to collect my thoughts, Terri waited with the patience of a kindergarten teacher. As I turned toward her, I noticed that she had laid both of her hands flat on the table, as if she was bracing for impact. Pausing for verbal running room, I began to describe the couch incident.

"What do you mean, you didn't recognize me?" she said. "How did I look different?"

"The longer that I stared at you, the more your facial features seemed changed."

> People with MS cognitive symptoms often show no obvious signs of the difficulties or a disability. It is a cruel illusion that can be explained through sharing your MS experience.

She appeared to be uncomfortable. She pushed her hardwood chair slightly away from the table and sat up straight. When the phone rang, neither of us reacted to it, not even by looking at the caller ID. I reached over and turned off the volume on the answering machine.

"Dr. Matthais said this is another type of delay in the processing of recollection, similar to the driving incident," I said, "except it happens with recognizing people, too. It passed within minutes, and I didn't even want to tell you about it; what would be the point?"

"But you said that it happened other times, too?" She wanted and deserved a full explanation.

"You know when we're all leaving in the morning," I continued, "and sometimes I stop before kissing you and jokingly say, 'Wife, right?' Well, that's actually not a joke."

"Meaning what?" she said.

"Sometimes everything is so confusing that I question what I'm doing. It's not as if I don't know what is supposed to happen, but when there's a piece suddenly missing, everything seems out-of-place."

"Why didn't you say something sooner?" Terri said.

"The kids were there or the time wasn't right, and frankly, I didn't know what this was, much less what to say about it."

"And that's what happened on the couch?" she said.

"Yes, but that time was prolonged and a little spooky. The harder I tried to snap out of it, the more I was drawn into an awareness of the change. It's not something that you can anticipate or control."

The kitchen was quiet. She interlaced her fingers and gently rested them on the table, as she absorbed my account of the incident and the doctor's analysis. Then, she adjusted herself again, easing back in the chair and stretching out her legs.

"And this is MS, again?" she said, finally.

"Matthais says it's another classic form of MS. It's not surprising that no one talks about it. Who would?"

"You had to ask me if I was *your wife*?" She smiled at the thought and tried to imitate my tone of voice when asking the ridiculous question.

"It was the quickest thing I could think of to slow down and check the moment." Suddenly, the delay technique seemed comical, and we both began to laugh.

"Fortunately, you agreed with me each time I asked. Come to think of it, I was never prepared for you to answer 'no.' Thanks for being consistent."

Laughter brings people together.

"So, is there anything we should do about this?" said Terri.

"Other than talking about it, there is probably nothing we can do. But as long as you asked, maybe you should sit in on my next appointment and hear it straight from Dr. Matthais. She can explain it better than I can. Besides, the hospital cafeteria now serves Starbucks coffee."

That wasn't so bad. Talking to Terri about my recognition lapses was natural and easy. We would learn to handle this twist of MS together—remembering that a good hug is when both people are holding on together.

◆ ◆ ◆

"Daddy, can you please brush my hair," said Meredith, pointing at the red brush perched on the corner of the bathroom pedestal sink. "I'm done with breakfast." Her 5-year-old blonde's waves of hair showed the tangled signs of sleep, tussled by a bed lined with stuffed animals. There were dozens upon dozens, and she not only knew the name of each cuddly face, but also the name of the store where the "friend" had been "found" and whether it had been a cash or Visa purchase. She didn't forget any details.

"Sure," I answered, "just stand in front of me and hold your head still so I can see you straight on in the mirror." As I searched for the part down the middle of her hair, I smiled back at the reflection of my daughter's face. Would I remember who she was tonight, when I tucked her into bed?

"Daddy, would you please help me with my spelling," said Meredith, later that evening.

"What did she just ask me?" I said to Terri.

Meredith had spoken clearly, but her sentences hit me like jumbled, three-word phrases. It was as if the information had entered my brain in slow-moving bursts that were not connected. The simple interaction felt like being asked an overlapping, four-part question while also trying to talk on the phone.

Meredith shifted her gaze from me to Terri, and then back again.

"She asked if you would quiz her on the spelling list," said Terri.

Everything was out of sync with no coherent reference point. A year earlier, I might have lashed out verbally when a demand was made. Unexpected disorientation is certainly frustrating, but reacting calmly is crucial. A practical way to respond is to act like one of those battery-operated cars that blindly hits a wall, but then knows to back up slightly and move in a different direction.

"Sure," I said, "let's go sit somewhere quiet so we can concentrate." Meredith grabbed her backpack and headed toward the living room.

My lapse was certainly innocent enough for Meredith to understand and deal with. It didn't require me to strike out, leaving her sad about asking me a simple question that I couldn't immediately answer. There is never a reason to let things develop to the point at which anger is triggered.

The front cover of the October–December 2003 issue of *InsideMS* depicted the very green and destructive *Incredible Hulk*. The lead article dealt with managing anger, a common reaction to the difficulties presented by MS. The useful discussion reminded me that there are always lighter ways to deal with stress. Anger had never benefited anyone in my family. Humor is the real superhero when battling MS. By learning to understand and sometimes defuse my own anger with laughter, my family has not become collateral damage in my struggle.

Coping with potential stress in social situations is similar to learning to deal with physical exacerbations. The thinking fatigue of MS is no different than the sudden onset of numbing weakness in legs. People with MS can have their energy and ability to concentrate depleted with little or no notice. They are vulnerable to experiencing information overload and need to avoid stacking up too many details to be processed at the same time. It is a matter of eliminating distractions and avoiding waves of extra information that pull thoughts off their original course. No piling on of tasks is allowed. It's another way of saying, "One thing at a time, or please give me a moment."

In addition to avoiding information overload, my family has learned to avoid stacking our schedules with a succession of tasks and other "mobile commotion," unless there is a true need to do so. When the opportunity is merely to chase from one activity to another and then back to another, the simple answer is, "No, thank you."

The visual use of Post-Its™ is a way to avoid the thinking congestion. If I didn't write it down when it occurred to me, the idea might not be there when I needed it. There were running lists for the hardware and grocery stores, and the daily "Do this stuff today while you are out there" list. Without the ability to quickly record points of reference, most of the information disappeared beyond recall.

Drifting along at an MS pace sometimes means, "No phone calls tonight"—or telling people, "Please don't ask me to listen to something while I'm driving and searching for parking." It may be too much to process right now, so relax and let it calmly roll by.

◆ ◆ ◆

"Did you hear what you just said?" said Terri, gently pulling me out into the hallway. "You said the word 'book' when you probably meant to say 'shirt,' when you were talking to Lauren about cleaning up her room. It made no sense, but I didn't want to point it out in front of the girls."

"I didn't notice anything odd," I said.

"I always hesitate to bring this kind of thing up, but I've noticed you doing it more often lately, saying one word when you mean to say another."

This was a switch from my usual struggle to find words during conversation. The trouble with word switching is that others may notice it before you are aware of it. Terri normally didn't have to point out an MS event, but being totally oblivious to this one, I was grateful that she was the first person to mention it. I assumed that my internal confusion was somewhat private, and, for the most part, unnoticeable to others. But, if I'm not aware of what I'm saying, then this changes everything. *Am I repeating myself or just speaking nonsense?*

"My speech is not matching my intention," I told Dr. Matthais. "It's fine if people correct me, but they probably won't. They'll just walk away thinking the worst, and my relationships will suffer." *Was I going to lose my ability to talk to other people?*

"Don't you have an appointment with Dr. Thomas coming up?"

"Yes, in two weeks. He's going to review my recent MRI scans. I received a call about the results, and was told that there was another new lesion, but it's nothing big to worry about. My need for mental space to collect my thoughts before speaking seems to be getting greater. I also seem to need more space between me and other cars when I'm driving."

"Are you concerned about having an accident?" said Dr. Matthais.

"No; my reaction time still seems okay. However, when difficulties with vision, balance, and confused direction hit all at once, I find myself talking out loud to stay focused. Actually, Terri does a lot of the driving now."

"By the time you meet with Dr. Thomas," said Dr. Matthais, "he and I will have talked about your MRI images and any next steps that might be necessary."

Fortunately, there were other "steps" available, whatever they might be, rather than merely accepting the inevitable from MS and taking the hits. Life could definitely be much worse. *This is not Alzheimer's*, I reminded myself.

The day before my appointment with Dr. Thomas, I found myself standing in the kitchen trying to hang up the phone on a cabinet door. It was too ridiculous to mention, but the phone would not work that way, and my brain *should* not!

"Terri has probably noticed my mistakes in conversation the most," I said to Dr. Thomas. "The thought just stops, I lose the word, and the concept of what I was saying is gone."

"Both your speech and listening capacity can be affected by MS, and your ability to quickly turn around the information is slowed."

He pointed at a small, new lesion on my MRI image, but he was unable to draw a connection between the small white mark and my misuse of words.

"There is something else that I would like to you consider," he said.

He had apparently already spoken with Dr. Matthais about my concerns. He told me about an encouraging new study demonstrating that Aricept®, a medication used to treat Alzheimer's patients, had shown the potential to improve memory in MS patients. *Would this translate into better verbal fluency and recognizing familiar faces and locations?* I wondered.

The medications used for Alzheimer's may also have the potential to improve memory in people with MS.

A larger study with Aricept® was beginning, with the goal of determining its safety and potential benefits for MS patients. However, it was still too early to be sure of any benefits. *Maybe they need volunteers for their study*, I thought.

Dr. Thomas handed me some printed materials about Aricept®. "Read up on the research, and I'll talk to Dr. Matthais about starting you on Aricept®," he said.

The recommendation to try Aricept® was on the cutting edge of treatment for MS cognitive symptoms, and I felt fortunate to be living at a time when so much medical knowledge was available. Aricept® might be able to save pieces of my daily functioning, so it was worth considering. It offered another opportunity to do something about MS.

Tips for Living

Avoiding Confusion

◆ Tell the people you care about, and who care about you, that you are having difficulties in thinking and focusing so that they can understand and support you.

◆ Identify the time of day when your ability to concentrate is best, and plan demanding mental activities for that time.

◆ Continue your prescribed medication and other therapies. See your doctors and therapists regularly to discuss the effectiveness of your therapies and whether any changes are needed.

◆ Limit the amount of information to be processed at any one time.

◆ Participate in one conversation at a time. Let people know that you might become confused if everyone talks at once.

◆ Keep your commitments to a tolerable level. Coordinate family schedules carefully. Surviving a crammed calendar gives only a false sense of accomplishment.

◆ Learn to say *no* to demands by others for your time and attention.

◆ Use visual cues, such as Post-Its™, to avoid confusion. Put them in obvious places where you will see them often.

◆ Keeping a daily written list is another good way to stay on track. As discussed in Chapter 8, a handheld electronic memory device can be quite useful.

◆ Strive for balance in your daily life.

◆ Do not make significant decisions when you feel fatigued or overwhelmed.

◆ Shift to a different word or expression when you can't think of a specific word. Allow yourself to rephrase.

◆ Repeat details to yourself and close family members, saying them out loud for confirmation.

◆ Keep a journal to record your feelings and ways of dealing with MS.

◆ Schedule a time for stretching and exercising your body, especially those areas that appear to be slowing down. The exhilaration of physical activity will stimulate your cognitive functioning.

CHAPTER ELEVEN

Come Out, Come Out, Wherever You Are

"That's an intriguing question," said the person who answered my telephone call to the Multiple Sclerosis Education Network. "If you can hold for a minute, I'll place you in line for it to be answered on the air." My heart started pounding. I had never before spoken on a live nationwide program about anything, much less MS. The program topic was the management of cognitive and emotional issues in MS, but other than questions about forgetfulness, the discussion had not delved into mind twists such as the ones I had experienced. Somebody needed to ask whether it was more common among MS patients than was generally understood. When she put me on the air, I explained briefly about getting lost while driving and my recognition difficulties.

"That sounds horrible!" said the program moderator. Then he turned the question over to a neurologist for a more clinical response. The neurologist calmly confirmed that my experiences were common in MS and that I was definitely not alone in dealing with mental challenges. Nevertheless, I was still shocked by the moderator's reaction, wondering whether his response was typical. If so, then it's no wonder why some MS patients avoid telling others about their cognitive difficulties.

That which remains hidden will continue to cause suffering.

After retiring from the practice of law, I would occasionally stop by the office to have lunch with my former colleagues. One day, as I waited in the reception area, Paulette, the receptionist spoke to me in a subdued voice: "Can I ask you a personal question?" She glanced down the hall as if trying to avoid detection.

"Sure, as long as I don't have to write any letters." She ignored my sarcasm and stared at me as if she was scanning for insight.

"Are you dying?" She hesitantly focused on my eyes as she spoke, perhaps looking for an answer that she might not want to hear. The phone began to ring, but she let another secretary pick up the call. She was serious about her question.

"Not that I know of," I said. "Why would you think that?"

"I've noticed that you've lost a lot of weight and you don't look so good," she said. (Steroids and the side effects of other medications can cause weight loss.)

"A friend of mine has MS, and she told me about a person who recently died from MS. And I wondered about you, especially since you retired."

"When you present it that way, the signals might suggest dying. MS has been tough, but I'm O.K., probably better off than other people with more fatal diseases."

"You're telling me the truth, right?"

"People typically don't die from multiple sclerosis."

Her sincere question, along with the radio moderator's shocked comment, served as benchmarks for a misconstrued and largely underestimated disease that few people talked about. The general misconceptions about MS are only the tip of the iceberg—considering how many people do not understand its far-reaching cognitive impact. Answers are available, but people must first be able to ask the questions. How many other physicians like Dr. Lazow will leave their patients in the dark about the cognitive aspects of MS?

The Wisconsin Chapter of the NMSS asked me to speak at their Newly Diagnosed Educational Series. It was an opportunity to provide practical information about the real challenges of MS as well as a chance to dispel myths. Walking into a room filled with a dozen people who had been newly diagnosed with MS, each sitting with a support person, felt like being on the inside of a fish tank and looking out at apprehensive customers.

They wanted to know everything about MS, yet not know. The more they understood, the more they might recognize symptoms in themselves, and this was a bit frightening. They were interested in knowing my personal story, which covered the continuum from diagnosis through assisting the MS Society. Speaking with other MS patients is always comfortable for me, so I shared my experiences and answered their concerns, including questions about the cognitive symptoms that had led to my retirement.

"That sounds exactly like what's screwing me up, too!" said Mark, a man with a dark-gray beard. "Sometimes, I just can't think straight, and I get upset with everybody. So, that's MS? My doctor is nice, but he doesn't say or do anything about it." Mark was obviously frustrated, but he smiled and seemed relieved to hear that his "thinking" problems were real.

Keep asking questions until you understand and are satisfied with the answers.

"Yes, it definitely can be MS," I said. "Although cognitive problems are discussed in the MS literature, they are not the first symptoms that draw attention. I'm not a doctor, so the best thing to do is call the MS Society. Ask them to send you information about the thinking and emotional difficulties of MS. Then, make a list of the problems that you experience and take it to your neurologist. Get your questions answered! If your neurologist doesn't seem to understand or care about your concerns, then consider finding another doctor. The MS Society can give you a list of neurologists with experience in treating multiple sclerosis."

"It makes me feel better to know that I'm not just freaking out." Mark said, looking at the other people in the room for confirmation.

"Maybe MS has something to do with my lack of concentration," said a young woman, who was wearing a Wisconsin Badgers football shirt. "I'm so easily thrown off in a conversation and forget what I was saying. My doctor thinks I'm too stressed, but she didn't say it was MS." Others in the group began to nod their heads in agreement. As I continued to discuss possible ways to find information about cognitive symptoms, several of the participants began to take notes.

"You may only get one good chance to take care of your MS," I said. "So don't sell your treatment short if you're not getting your questions answered. This is not a 'little cold,' it's multiple sclerosis!"

Even with these newly diagnosed patients, cognitive symptoms had already struck a loud, mysterious chord in their lives. Although the discussion may have confirmed and alleviated some of their initial questions, I left the session concerned about the level of treatment they might receive from their doctors and the reactions of friends.

Writing a book seemed more necessary than ever before, so I continued to keep a written record of my cognitive challenges as well as my encounters with other patients. Retirement had given me the time to write, even considering the inconsistent pace of my mental recall and processing of ideas. It would take time, but I would finish the project despite MS.

As a Peer Supporter at the MS Society, I had access to a library of MS-related books, videos, and other publications; I studied these materials in between answering telephone calls. The reading and conversations provided me with a wealth of information to address the multifaceted questions of MS patients. The callers varied from individuals who were newly diagnosed to those who have had MS for many years. We were as different as passengers on a crowded train, yet we were all traveling in the same direction.

"Would you be willing to go with us to the state capitol for our first MS legislative initiative?" said Renee Vandlik, the Advocacy Manager for the Wisconsin Chapter of the NMSS. "Your personal story and your experience as a Peer Supporter would be very useful in speaking to legislators about supporting our MS-related concerns."

She didn't have to ask me twice, and I still had the necessary suits and ties.

Well armed with briefing materials, our group of MS advocates invaded the state capitol in Madison, meeting with legislator after legislator. Among other things, we requested funding for a program that would provide MRI scans for indigent women. When MS patients are diagnosed and begin using medication sooner rather than later, they have a better chance of slowing the progression of the disease, all to the benefit of their families and society. For every woman who was fortunate to have their diagnosis of MS confirmed as early as possible, I envisioned that it might mean one less person being seated in a wheelchair or thinking that they were losing their mind.

It was a record-budget-deficit year and a miserable time to approach the government with a request for new funding, but our efforts paid off, and the legislation was eventually passed, funded, and signed by the Governor.

Next, I was asked to join a small Wisconsin Chapter contingency that was traveling to Washington, D.C., for the NMSS Annual Public Policy Conference. I felt honored to be included in this direct lobbying of our Wisconsin senators and congressmen.

"Don't forget to bring your walking stick," said Terri. "There's bound to be a lot of walking, in between the cab and Metro rides."

"It's already collapsed and packed," I said.

Airport security took my nail clippers the last time I flew. I hope they don't confiscate my stick because of the brass handle.

Although I had been to Washington, D.C., many times and was familiar with the city, I was acutely aware that I sometimes get lost in my own neighborhood. Imagine the horror of becoming disoriented while switching subway cars, but with my cell phone and PDA full of key telephone numbers in my briefcase, I felt safe. I would certainly avoid being alone in unfamiliar settings. My father dropped me off at the airport, where I was met by the other advocates. As long as I stuck with them while traveling through airports and from Senate office to Senate office, I would be fine.

"You have MS?" said Senator Herb Kohl.

People with MS sometimes show no obvious symptoms; they look "just fine."

His stunned reaction to my disclosure, as well as the reactions of the other legislative staffers, was typical, even though they each seemed to have a friend or close relative with MS. More than 10,000 people in Wisconsin have MS, and the legislators are aware of the numbers. We were definitely within their represented district, and our message was well received and supported. It was the best kind of political exchange to directly advocate for a nonprofit health-related cause.

Lobbying on behalf of the NMSS, especially as a volunteer, took the fight against MS to a new level. We were not the same as the other lobbyists who passed us in the halls, many of whom were pushing for a measure to protect a business interest or financial profit. Our efforts were about garnering support for changes that would help people we would never meet but with whom we shared a common adversary.

"Could you write something for the *MS Connections* newsletter about your success with the advocacy program?" said Renee Vandlik.

"I think it would mean a lot to the advocacy program if other people in the state saw what we accomplished this past year."

The newsletter was routinely mailed out to all of the Chapter members and was read by countless family members, neurologists, and other people who were in touch with the mission of the MS Society.

"Yes; whatever it takes to get people involved." As long as I didn't have a crushing deadline and could write at my own pace, I would be able to do it. Being an attorney had been a purposeful trade, but it paled in comparison to writing about engaging volunteers to help others deal with MS.

"Would you be willing to write a story for *Facilitator Flash*, our Self-Help Group newsletter?" said Diane Baughn. "With your experience as an advocate in Madison, and now in Washington, you could tell others how to get involved in supporting MS legislation."

It sounded like a natural extension of what I was already doing to get the word out, so I agreed. Writing about MS was easy because I wrote from the heart of my own experience.

This phase of my volunteer activities culminated in my being awarded the NMSS Wisconsin Chapter's 2003 Outstanding Volunteer Award, but I considered it as further motivation. The award represented only the beginning of my efforts to reach out to those silent people with MS who were experiencing cognitive difficulties.

And I didn't have to do it alone. Although our "Summit Team" was a rookie team for the MS-Walk, I was humbled by the turnout of 43 family members and friends, as well as their financial contributions from across the country. The Summit Team not only represented the name of our street, Summit Avenue, it symbolized how far we would take our effort to fight MS. Together with Terri and our girls, we constituted the largest individual team in the Wisconsin MS-Walk and, after our first 2 years, we have raised over $12,000 for MS educational programs and research. Given the opportunity to join in the fight against MS, people will "do something" about it.

As I continued volunteering in a variety of capacities, I increasingly turned my attention to writing this book and, as it neared completion, I began to reflect upon what I was sharing and how it might have an impact on my family and any lingering issues of self-esteem

I might have. Then I recalled the comments of Colleen Kalt, the President of the Wisconsin Chapter of the MS Society, who had enthusiastically endorsed my writing project: "Are you prepared to open yourself up so completely?" she said. "I give you a lot of credit for writing about the cognitive challenges of MS. Your book will help countless people."

I knew she was right to ask me whether I was ready to be seen in what might be considered an unflattering light, but there was no other way to do it. There is no pride in admitting that MS has affected my ability to think clearly, but discussing it was not new. I was determined to stay focused on the MS Society's credo: *I have MS, but it doesn't have me.*

Through education, MS can be fought face-to-face.

The best hope of slowing the potential cognitive challenges of MS is to educate people and encourage them to take off the *mask* and not waste their precious energy hiding their mental stumbling. Through education, MS can be fought face-to-face. Although early diagnosis and treatment can slow the progression of symptoms, unfortunately many people hide their mental confusion and remain silent. They don't believe that it's real or that it's MS. A person must be able to identify and come to grips with their mental difficulties before they can accurately describe them to their doctor. Only then can they accept beneficial medication and learn how to compensate.

Although neurologists are generally aware of the classic symptoms of cognitive impairment, many of them miss the connection to MS. They assume the ability to think is not directly affected by the disease. In fact, a neurologist's typical examination of an MS patient may not even include questions about cognitive difficulties, but includes only physical symptoms. Without comments by the patient, mental disorientation may be missed and be left untreated.

The stigma attached to mental disease is real. Within that labeled reality is the fear of becoming less than a *normal* person. The fear of the label is also real. Aversion to being branded with an MS cognitive deficiency is inherent throughout the diagnosis process. A deep exploration of the initial signs, discovery, and emerging "thinking" changes is vital. Many people with MS believe that they are alone in facing these challenges. "Cognitive Difficulties" must be more than just a label on a patient's file. Encouraging complete disclosure is necessary to understand and put an end to the nightmare of mental confusion from MS.

◆ ◆ ◆

"Come out, come out, wherever you are!" we yelled in our childhood game of hide-and-seek. However, despite the numbers of people who call the MS Society for information, many others remain unaware that an explanation and treatment is available to sustain them through their most mind-bending cognitive challenges. The very nature of volunteering is inherently fulfilling. It creates something positive in the midst of an otherwise devastating situation. On an "Oprah" scale of reaching out, I decided that writing a book would be the best vehicle to inform the MS community about the potential cognitive dysfunctions associated with MS.

As a Peer Supporter for the Wisconsin Chapter of the MS Society, I have been fortunate to have the opportunity to assist hundreds of people with disabilities. Individuals beset with medical and personal challenges reach out to Peer Supporters—strangers who have been there and understand their suffering. They deserve accurate information, direction, and encouragement.

Sharing my life with others, even with all of my unseemly cognitive and physical challenges, only affirms that *I am amazingly blessed with purpose and still in a good place*. I have been blessed with the opportunity to help others understand MS and learn to cope. It is all about listening to humanity, sharing, and encouraging people with MS, to keep moving through life with it even if only one moment at a time.

Tips for Living

- ◆ Find the corners of the world that hold meaning for you and use your skills to further improve them.
- ◆ Join your local chapter of the NMSS and learn all you can from the available publications. Participate in fundraising for MS research and broader education.
- ◆ Share your expertise to benefit other patients and their families and friends.

◆ Reach out through volunteering and share your spirit and life experiences. It's a useful and engaging way to keep your cognitive skills sharp, without the stressful burden of maintaining employment.

◆ After you have established a personal method of symptom management, consider sharing what you have learned with other MS patients. Your symptoms and coping techniques may seem obvious or unique, but there are many others who could benefit from your insight.

◆ By supporting others, you support yourself.

CHAPTER TWELVE

In the Game

Where are they—our girls? Lauren was sitting next to me in the front passenger seat of my VW and Meredith was behind her, alone in the backseat. Meredith's school lunch bag was resting in the bottom of her blue-flowered backpack and she was concerned about smashing her peanut butter sandwich and grapes under a history book. Without any warning, they were gone and I was alone in the car. I glanced over my shoulder to see an empty backseat. Did I forget to pick them up, or worse, did I leave them someplace and drive away? The girls are now 15 and 12 years old and I just can't imagine the fear and puzzled looks that they are sharing with each other. My mind can't think clearly about their location and where I am going—driving into an MS cognitive nightmare.

Getting into an accident would only make matters worse and a kind horn toot snapped me to the reality of the green light. I turned the car past the Mobil gas station on the corner and pulled to the curb behind the station's parked tow truck. This was Downer Avenue and our home was just one mile down the road. That much I knew, but my mind was desperately flailing like a drowning swimmer. Alright, where are they? Where are they supposed to be at this moment? Think! This moment was real, but I had frequently been here before and learned from it—be safe, remain calm, and ignore any panic. This was not the missing-person scene from the Harrison Ford movie, *Frantic*. It began to dawn on me that I must have skipped a step in the morning routine and that they are waiting to be picked up by me—somewhere. But where? Relax, think calmly, and let it come back!

> When suddenly confounded about traveling or direction, immediately place yourself in a safe position, then deal with the loss of presence.

Like a secret password through an invisible speakeasy door, this is the most common question that I am asked. The person may soften their voice perceiving that it may be a sensitive subject for me, but then frankly ask whether I still have those "lost moments." Similar to many people with MS, I still arrive unannounced in the thick MS cognitive forest sometimes not recognizing where I am going, who I am talking to, or forgetting the next line of what I was going to say? Things like that. This acknowledgment is emotionally leveling, realizing that MS has permanently tinkered with the connections in my mind. Dwelling there offers no purpose or direction.

Although the answer to the repeated question hasn't improved for me during the past several years, I am better prepared to deal with it. Almost every day I catch myself mentally stumbling to grasp a point of what I intended to do. Whether in a conversation, walking into a room, grabbing the phone, or getting in the car, there may be a hitch in my line of thinking that frequently halts me from the next step.

While the mental gaps still occur and surprise me like a pop quiz, they have not seemed to progress in intensity, nor have they gone away. Suddenly, uncomplicated thoughts can appear as unintelligible as uncharted mountain ranges. Rather than deciding to beat my head against the rock walls, I have found that it is far more productive to discuss these cognitive disconnections and share what has helped me cope with them. I'm grateful for the opportunities offered to me to participate in the MS cognitive discussion and I have been overwhelmed by the welcoming response.

During the past several years, I have gladly accepted invitations from the MS community to participate in book signings and other MS presentations. After taking a break from my brief reading at the NMSS Advocacy Conference at the Hilton in Washington, D.C., I was guided to a book signing table outside of the cavernous conference room. I slid my cane under the chair and reached for the glass of water waiting for me on the table.

"We have copies of both of your books," said Kim Kinner, "but more of the first one." Kim was the Director of Community Education and Outreach for the Wisconsin Chapter of the NMSS and often assisted me with book signings at MS events. "Hope your hand doesn't cramp." I was more concerned about my cane jutting out from under the table and tripping someone. Kim had already ripped open the cardboard boxes of books and neatly streamlined the stacks of each book for quick signing. "There were over 300 people in that room," she mentioned, "so this should be interesting if we run out of books." We did. It wasn't the first or last time that the hunger for MS cognitive discussion showed itself by the devouring of piles of both books that I had written about the subject.

As the line moved by, one of the conference attendees stood in front of me with a couple of copies of each book in her hands. She was professionally dressed, wearing a blue jacket with a NMSS embossed name tag pinned to the lapel.

"Jeffrey, thank you so much for your writing and reading for us today. These copies are for our Chapter library to lend to our Self-Help groups," she said, as she placed them in front of me to sign. "When I read your first book I learned so much about MS cognitive problems and was wondering"—she leaned further over the table—"do you have those memory moments during your presentations?" Was it so obvious? I wondered.

"All the time," I answered and slowly nodded my head. "I rely heavily on my notes to guide me, but I get easily lost and never seem to cover all of the material on the paper. That is why I like taking questions, it helps me fill in the areas that I probably lost"—I placed my finger to my mouth—"shhhh, but don't tell anyone." She smiled and seemed to understand that I preferred not to take myself too seriously. "Hopefully, people take home some meaningful discussion about MS cognitive difficulties and explore strategies for themselves."

"They're already out of books!" said Meredith, as she smiled, and sat down in a chair beside me and kicked off her sandals. She was definitely comfortable at these signing events and I was grateful that she enjoyed the experience of meeting people from all over the country. During book signings, Meredith enjoyed being asked to sign her name next to my illegible retired-lawyer signature. Lauren and Terri *rotated with Meredith, traveling with me as a caregiver to ensure that I get on the right airplane and show up at the correct hotel. This sets my mind at ease to concentrate on my presentation notes and without one of them beside me to fill in my mental blanks, I am at risk that my "loss of presence" would simply become—lost.*

> Relying on a trusted person is enabling.

Fall leaves were dropping from a tree near the tow truck and were blowing across the sidewalk, collecting against a wire mesh fence. My mind persistently echoed: Where are the girls? The navy blue tow truck seemed ready for action, but unfortunately, it couldn't take me where I needed to go.

Wait for it. It tends to come back much easier if I let the thoughts go. What seems like 10 minutes of torturous waiting for reality to click in may only be a minute or less. I let my mind wander to other short concerns: my car needed to be washed, who the Packers are playing on Sunday, and returning library books. Dave, the radio announcer on 96.5 WKLH, announced that it was 8:25 on Monday morning and that the news update was coming up at the half hour.

Click. The clear reality was that Lauren and Meredith were already at school. Earlier that morning, I had dropped each of them off at their different schools, but I could not access the recent memory of it as I was driving home. The relief from a nightmare doesn't remove the moments of terror you experience during the disorientation, but buying time and remaining calm can clear the mental fog—a dramatic reason why I could never be a doctor or an air-traffic controller, holding any position requiring mental consistency and a reliable functioning memory.

When I allowed myself a calm moment to realize that I was almost home, alone in the car, and that morning classes for both girls had already started, then I recalled already taking them to school. The missing piece of my morning was always there, but I had difficulty accessing it with added stress. Once calm and undistracted, my thoughts seemed to clear like a lens coming slowly into focus.

It may have been confusing for me, since Lauren started high school and Meredith was still attending a middle school, but it all came back to me once I stopped fighting and taking empty swings of frustration.

It may be especially difficult to withhold primordial feelings of fear or panic, but I know that if I calm my senses, then I can tap down the cognitive twister. After a tornado strikes, there is news footage showing the extreme damage leaving viewers to wonder how the devastation will be cleaned up. By avoiding panic in the midst of the MS cognitive twister, I evade the wreckage of my own collateral damage.

> Remaining calm when mentally lost allows the thought to return.

How could I not remember where I had dropped off the girls? A 10,000-piece puzzle may seem obvious to assemble when you are looking at the finished product, but not so much when all you can see is the pile when it is dumped out of the box. It can take a great deal of self-discipline and patience to work through the wreckage of pieces to sort out a clear picture. Tipping over the table is never a way to assemble a puzzle. MS holds many puzzles, but it is clear to see that since my diagnosis in 1996, numerous and varied teams of individuals have successfully put some of the pieces together. The multifaceted MS community contributes their talents to raise funds and awareness for vital studies, while researchers receive funding to discover a better treatment. Each person pops in a crucial piece to solve the MS puzzle, and together, we will all see the complete picture.

What If?

The current sad truth is that there is still no cure for MS, yet, nor an ability to anticipate its disabling fallout with reliable accuracy. On the other hand, MS will only go away through our common efforts to support research and education. In the meantime, I welcome improved therapies that slow the progression of MS while I learn how to better cope with the parts of my mind and body that have been compromised. It is a different kind of endurance skill and one that is measured not by gaining great speed or strength, but by seeking another part of your existence to compensate for what was lost. With that awareness in your pocket, learn to keep moving and continue to adjust to whatever MS tosses your way.

If you tend to lose mental placement of known locations and directions, then you may need to back up the details on a handheld electronic device or just print the information, prior to departing.

If you have difficulty explaining MS cognitive difficulties to your significant other, a family member, or friend, then share a copy of this book or an MS cognition brochure from a known MS organization. Don't duck out on the conversation. Instead, invite a review of on-point published information, along with a third-party medical or counseling professional who understands the full impact of MS and cognition.

If you are concerned that vital pieces of your calendar or financial information may be mentally obscured, then identify a trusted individual and explain to them (in writing too) where and how these details are stored for practical reference. It is beyond my abilities to DVR the most confounded moments in my MS life, freezing the loss of presence and crucial information, enabling me to replay it over again for considered decision making. Give yourself the calm reassurance that important details will not be lost because you have already ensured that a trusted person is your backup for these details. It may be best to do this far in advance of MS interference, when life seems calm and understandable, rather than when you feel pressured to make a vital decision or recall needed information. For many, that may mean now.

If you want to avoid feeling that you are shunning contact and moving from one isolated island to another, then be open to sharing descriptions of your life-grounding mental fog. Arm dear friends and family with the available scientific facts about MS cognitive difficulties and disability, preparing them to assist you through those instances where your thought processes are blurred. Educating them up front regarding your jammed thinking functions may be the best method for them to back you up with kind understanding. It's what you would do for each of them if the shoes were reversed. Wouldn't you want to help them in an informed and useful manner?

A "Safety Person"

It is unreasonable to expect understanding from others if you haven't provided them with the insight into your frequently obscured perspective. The best of intentions won't really be that useful.

A "safety person" is qualified by your sharing MS cognitive information with them, including attending medical appointments, reading
MS cognitive brochures, and Web sites, and participating in cognition
conferences. The tools for an informed "safety person" are readily
available, but don't wait for these opportunities to find you. Reading
and sharing this book and my other publication, *Mental Sharpening Stones: Manage the Cognitive Challenges of Multiple Sclerosis*
(Demos Medical Publishing, 2008), is certainly a good start to assembling your informed MS cognitive team. Engage in the conversation
and allow it to work for you.

> MS is best handled with support and not in isolation.
> Don't go alone.

The concept of a "sure thing" is understood by most people. It is a
guarantee that something that is desired or anticipated will happen.
No question that you may count on it and obviously, I am not refer-
ring to sports, politics, or stocks. When listening to the words of the
Pledge of Allegiance or A Psalm of David, you can recite the phrasing because maybe you have done so thousands of times and it has
deep meaning for you. "*I pledge allegiance to the flag....*" If you were
asked to join in with others reading these words, it would sound familiar and touch that part of your heart. "*The Lord is my Shepherd,
I shall not want....*" The private sentiments of those words belong to
you and if they were gone when you reached for them, it would feel
like a personal theft.

My family is Jewish. My father, who is still living, and his parents
were survivors of the Warsaw Ghetto. Despite Hitler's efforts, I am
aware that I am here only because of their instincts, blessings, and a
little luck outrunning the Gestapo. Practically everyone they knew
(family and friends) and whatever they held in the poverty of the
ghetto was liquidated by the Nazis. With this family history always
in mind, I intend that my prayers, whether routine or associated with
a special holiday or occasion, be valued beyond the words on the
page. Perhaps like many of those who attend church every Sunday
morning, my family makes a real effort to regularly attend Shabbat

services on Saturday mornings, and like many others, we end up sitting in the same seats. I have listened to and recited the prayers since I was a little boy and whether following the right-to-left Hebrew in the prayer book or reciting by heart, I felt confident that I knew my stuff.

> MS cognitive disruption can strike at well-known information without notice.

One of those daily prayers is the *Amidah*, and when the congregation rose to their feet with prayer books in hand and began to chant in unison, *Barukh atah Adonai*, I glanced to the top of the page to jumpstart reciting the words. It was all gone.

As my hand grabbed and pulled on the back of the burnt-orange cloth seat in front of me, Terri held my left elbow, giving me a boost to smoothly rise to my feet. The routine reminds me of a coach helping a player to his feet and saying, "Now get in there." Although I had stood up and was now leaning on the chair for balance, the movement failed to trigger my mind to join in the chanted words. Nothing. The congregation was on the next page and I screamed in my mind unsuccessfully to get in-sync, but then decided to mentally restart the prayer. Still nothing but frustration, and, now, I was completely lost in the Hebrew text. Terri noticed that I wasn't turning any pages and that I had remained silent.

"Everything alright?" she quietly asked and held my arm. The melodic murmur of the prayer rolled along without me as I felt my head slowly shake side-to-side. My left knee buckled and as I reached to grab the seat, the prayer book slipped from my hand and was caught between my thigh and the chair—saved from the carpeted floor. Without shifting my gaze from my shoes, I could sense that others turned toward my commotion.

"Just fine," I softly answered, "but I need to sit down." It didn't matter that sitting down during a standing prayer might draw more attention; I needed to recoup some composure. Either way I was going down. My choice was either sitting in the chair or hitting the ground. Without saying a word or requiring any explanation, Terri held her grip on my arm and eased me into my chair. Resting on the edge of the seat with my head slumped over the prayer book, I shifted to the English and read through a paragraph involving being sustained. Perfect.

My physical slip was public, but the lost prayer was private and painful. I would gladly exchange 100 physical hits for the one cognitive void, but I don't make these MS rules. When part of my body doesn't seem to function as it should, I can see it struggling. When my mind draws a blank, all I can sense is that there should be something there. When a routine thought is inaccessible, it feels like a piece of my mind is missing. Calmly releasing the panicked mental grip allows the cognitive piece to fit back into its slot, reclaiming my purpose and essence.

> Relaxing your thoughts allows them to naturally regroup and make sense out of simple confusion.

Fortunately for me, Terri is attuned to my weakened coordination or when my mind is locked out of the moment. She calmly notes my difficulties and avoids drawing attention to the impediment, while giving me the safe mental space to clear my puzzlement. Knowing that I feel more capable with a "safety person," I can then focus on: Accepting the difficulty, Better understanding what is occurring, and learning to Cope with it.

This simple **A-B-C** method is shared not as a means to ignore MS, but to remove any fear and learn that you have more to gain by gracefully moving forward with your life. When MS plays the role of the rude permanent guest in my life, it is helpful to rely on the **A-B-C** path. The "**A**" also reminds me to **A**pologize for my mental stumbles, rather than have friends or family be uncomfortable with my awkward lapses.

When Terri and I sat down for a holiday dinner with a large group of friends, I addressed the wife of a close friend as "Jamie." Since we were all sitting at the same long table with several other friends, they all clearly heard me. Terri grabbed my arm and with a forgiving smile, leaned into me.

"You mean Cathy, and not Jamie," she whispered. My eyes remained fixed on my plate and silverware, as I suddenly recalled that

I hadn't seen Jamie in 15 years, since her divorce from Travis. He had been married to Cathy for a couple of years and she was sitting across the table from me averting my gaze. A slice of turkey had just landed on my plate, resting under a blanket of gravy, flanked by green beans, and a warm dinner roll. So sad that I have come to envy a dead turkey, but I wanted to hide with it under the mountain of mashed potatoes.

My brain must have known that I hadn't mentioned or seen Jamie in 20 years, but I was unaware of the word switching. Terri has mentioned these instances to me in an effort to show the frequency and innocence of the misspoken word, but this unintentionally stung others. It is even more awkward when no one feels comfortable enough to point out one of my verbal switches, thinking it is best to not mention it. Our group of friends was silently forgiving, since I was quick to accept my switching of names and apologize for the embarrassing miscue. A great insult, confusion, and possibly a food fight were avoided, thanks to my "safety person."

> Trust a "safety person" to guide you toward a calm and rational explanation.

Despite any embarrassment, Terri knew how to gently correct my words, and I trusted that she would explain it to me later. It often feels as if my thoughts are jammed full and without any room for new discussion. Rather than sentencing myself to self-isolation, I am grateful to follow Terri's lead and timing, gracefully pulling away from awkward conversation-ending moments. Trusting her to set me straight without drama has been comforting, and I can only hope to return the blessing to her—times a thousand.

Tips for Living

- ◆ Trust what you have learned about yourself and MS to guide yourself through the most challenging MS cognitive incidents. MS cannot rewrite your personal history.
- ◆ While certainly many things may be worse than dealing with MS, don't dwell on the unknown as being inevitable.

- Neither your education nor the family and friends that surround you are erased. Hold them close, treasure their support, share your MS experience with them, and give yourself permission to focus on your health.
- Find your "safety person" and don't forget about the hugs.
- Consider the **A-B-C** method: **A**cknowledge, **B**etter understand, and **C**ope with MS setbacks, while not surrendering the future with family and friends. Holding this balance point is a source of constant adjustment in dealing with cognitive and physical challenges. You don't have the option to put one MS difficulty on hold while you deal with another.

Meredith, Terri, Jeffrey, and Lauren Gingold at the National Multiple Sclerosis Society's Annual Conference in Chicago, Illinois, after Jeffrey's induction to the NMSS 2010 Hall of Fame for Advocacy.

CHAPTER THIRTEEN

A Team Effort

It delivered as promised. For almost 8 years and on a weekly basis, Terri and I committed to the weekly routine of an IM injection of *Interferon beta 1a* directly into one of my thighs. The weekly injection ritual in the kitchen gave me an opportunity to watch reruns of every episode of *Frasier*, while I comfortably relied on Avonex® to slow the progression of my MS. Although I continued to wrestle with cognitive and physical impediments, mixed in with an overflowing bucket of pseudoexacerbations, Avonex® seemed to keep my MS from getting worse. MS never went away and I still battled confounded thinking, fatigue, numbness, and equilibrium difficulties, as well as the flu-like side effects from the medication.

That was the expected and somewhat reasonable part of the therapy package. Avonex® held the line against MS, and it allowed me to feel a bit in control, perhaps like a levee worker who runs back and forth between newly discovered leaks in the sea wall. The Avonex® wall held for me. With each injection of Avonex® into my body, I remained hopeful that there would be another "wall" available for me if this one ever became compromised.

Without Avonex® being available at the time of my MS diagnosis, my life would have been unquestionably at the total mercy of MS. There may be no way to measure how much MS would have devoured my life, but I am sure that without Avonex® it would have been far worse. Of course, when choosing a course of therapy each person with MS must make that informed determination for themselves, along with input from their support team. That was my choice and it worked for me.

After 7 years of Avonex® therapy, MS showed that it was not idle in my brain. As part of monitoring the progression of my MS, I had an MRI of my brain every 6 months. For the most part, the images remained similar to the prior set of images and lesions, depending on the slice of my brain caught in the scan. Dr. Thomas would always turn on the bright-light X-ray board and clip in the prior MRI images to compare with the current scan. Dr. Thomas had already read the report and seemed a bit more focused than usual on the typed detail in his hand. Once I exhausted comments dealing with the bizarre nature of seeing the pieces inside my own head, Dr. Thomas mentioned that there was a notable change in the scan. He waited for me to lift myself out of the chair and hobble over to the wall. Dr. Thomas drew my attention toward the lit scan and pointed toward a new bright spot on one of the images.

"When we compare this slice to a similar image from the last MRI," he noted, "we can see that this lesion wasn't there in the last set of slides, even with the contrast." He was wearing blue surgical scrubs and I decided that he had just come from somewhere sterile, rather than believing that my appointment would become invasive. Dr. Thomas explained that it would never be crystal clear whether a new lesion was forecasting another exacerbation or reflecting something that was currently in play, but it was disturbing to see. All of the denial and whiteout in the world cannot erase a lesion from an MRI scan of my brain.

"What am I doing wrong?" I asked. There were no guarantees for anyone living with MS, and I reminded myself that I have a progressive disease. "I have tried to cut away all the stressors in my life and maintain the Avonex® therapy, so where did this lesion come from?"

"What you may not be able to see is how the medication and adjustments in your life have probably prevented MS from getting much worse," said Dr. Thomas. "It is difficult to acknowledge a benefit from something that hasn't happened, but over the years using Avonex® has probably helped you." Dr. Thomas held his eye contact with me, as if looking for confirmation that I was attentive and understanding the conversation. He began to point at the MRI images and explained how the location of the lesions may be causing various difficulties that he observed in the neurological exam, but then I lost focus. I could only think about what was next for me.

"I know this is a lot of information to take in," continued Dr. Thomas, "but it doesn't mean that we should discount Avonex® at this point. None of the therapies can prevent all lesions and for you, an additional lesion does not by itself mean that Avonex® is not working." The best part of my doctor-patient relationship with Dr. Thomas is that he related to what I was thinking and not just because he could actually see into my brain. He understood me and knew that by itself, one more brain lesion would not redirect my course of treatment.

"This may not be a proper medical conclusion," I said, "but I still need two points to draw a straight line in another direction." Dr. Thomas knew my modus operandi for rationalizing a change of therapies. It wasn't a matter of simply switching needles.

"I agree and would feel stronger about exploring a change in medication if you were experiencing a significant exacerbation," said Dr. Thomas, "so I would like to do another MRI and blood labs before your next appointment and let's watch if anything else is happening." This made sense to me. If my MS was on the move, then I would have to adjust to that too. Leaving the medical clinic that morning, I had comfort in knowing that there was a game plan to deal with the bad lesion news. I may get comfortable with a pair of tennis shoes, but if they no longer fit or support me, then it may be time to look for a new pair.

Avonex® is an incredible therapy to control MS, but I had to consider that after 7 years, it might no longer be effective for my MS. Reflecting back on my first IM injection, I could never have foreseen how grateful I would feel for Avonex® being approved for use at the time of my diagnosis. Timing is everything. If it hadn't been available and selected as my first therapy stand against MS, I feel that my mind and body would have traveled much further down the disability road. Instead, I had taken informed measures to preserve my vitality until the next better therapy might be approved. For me, Avonex® remains the old friend that prevented my life ship from being sunk by incoming MS lesion torpedoes.

Perhaps the good news about having MS now and not 20 years ago is that there are even more options available for treatment. What hasn't changed is that after being educated regarding each course of treatment, each person with MS should still decide for themselves which therapy is best for them. Though I selected Avonex® as my first-line therapy doesn't mean that another person with MS should make the same decision. The choice of an MS therapy is personal and may be complicated by other factors that should be considered by an informed support team.

> Over time, the effectiveness of any MS medication may change and another medication may need to be considered.

When my next set of MRI images revealed yet another lesion, the decision to consider a therapy switch seemed appropriate and justified. Dr. Thomas, Terri, and I discussed other therapies that were available, and we decided that Rebif® would be a good step after being on Avonex® for so many years. I had read about Tysabri® and was excited to learn about its amazing success in studies for reducing new lesions, but it wasn't available at the time that I needed to make a change, so I would watch and wait for that prospect.

Using Rebif® would mean a *subcutaneous* injection three times a week, using a green autoinjector and rotating the sites on my body. Our cat, Mickey, knew that something different than the Avonex® routine was happening when she heard the test clicks from the autoinjector, causing her to flee the kitchen. This injection routine would be a little more complicated than Avonex®, mainly because of the frequency and also because each injection held the same "flu-like" symptoms for me, but now three times a week. While using Avonex® I adjusted my life to avoid demanding expectations during the hours after the injection, knowing that the balance of days until the next weekly injection would be manageable. If the physically pounded and mentally dragging feelings from each Rebif injection overlapped, then I wondered if I would ever experience moments of "normal" again. However, if Rebif® was the next effective step against a progressive MS, then fine, I would deal with it.

The Rebif® (Serono) staff was very supportive in their efforts to manage the side effects that I was experiencing. After several months on Rebif®, the dosage of the medication would be adjusted for me, searching for a tolerable level. Dr. Thomas was acutely aware of how the quality of my life was affected by the never-ending loop of flu-like symptoms, but I needed to see if Rebif® could pick up where Avonex® had left off. I don't walk out in the middle of movies or sporting events and Rebif® would be given time to show if it worked for me.

"Let's just put this on the table now, prior to seeing the next round of MRI results," I said to Dr. Thomas, as he began testing the diminished sensation in my left leg. "What are the options if despite being on Rebif® for months the next MRI also shows new brain lesions?" It was an anguishing question, but one that I preferred to address without being distressed by seeing more lesion images. With Dr. Thomas as a partner in the conversation, I felt assured that decisions would continue to be thoroughly considered and not an emotional reaction. Unfortunately, the next series of MRIs ended the discussion. Whether it was a result of the adjusted Rebif® dosage or a dozen other potential elements, another brain lesion spelled out MS progression for me. It was like watching a slow MS train wreck and I wanted to get off the line.

Tysabri®

No one could realistically pretend that the question wasn't on their mind. It loomed larger than a dozen 800-pound gorillas sitting in the corner, and there it would sit, until it was directly addressed. While I was speaking at an MS cognition educational conference in late 2010, the question came from the floor.

"Are you on any MS medication?" asked a lady wearing jeans and a Chicago Cubs T-shirt. She had finished her dinner and had pushed the plate toward the center of the table, clearing a spot for the conference materials and dessert. The event was casual, but her question was not and it cut to the heart of what is on the mind of many people with MS. As she handed the microphone back to the roving moderator, she glanced back and forth to another lady sitting next to her at the table. It wasn't clear who owned the question, but they both seemed hesitant to open the medication subject, staring at each other with an expression of "No, you ask him."

"I have been on Tysabri® for almost two years," I answered, "and on Avonex® for almost eight years prior to that." There were about 100 attendees at this conference and with that question and answer, all private table conversations ceased. They may have heard rumors, but I decided to share what I have learned and they could judge for themselves, be a little more informed.

While contemplating Tysabri® for myself, I encountered a report in the *International Journal of MS Care*, which noted that on April 29, 2009, Biogen Idec and Elan Corporation (manufacturer of Tysabri®) reported results from an ongoing 1-year longitudinal health outcomes study ($n = 1,275$) in which patients who received three infusions of Tysabri® (natalizumab) reported reduced fatigue and significant improvements in general and disease-specific measurements of quality of life. In reference to that report about MS and Tysabri®, it would be very easy for me to focus on five words: "significant improvements" and "quality of life." With that information in my pocket, I continued to study the use of Tysabri® and consider it for myself.

> When contemplating using an MS medication, do your research and ask relevant questions to be comfortable with your choice of therapy.

In November 2004, Tysabri was approved by the FDA for use by people with relapsing-remitting MS and early data reported that Tysabri® reduced by 68 percent MS relapse, compared with placebo, and cut by 42 percent the relative risk of disability progression. This spoke directly to me and I wanted to learn more about Tysabri®, its initial approval, and return to the market.

Tysabri® is given to a patient by IV infusion once every 4 weeks. According to the Biogen study, Tysabri® not only reportedly delays progression of MS but in some cases has shown improvement of disability. Unfortunately, there was a setback for those receiving Tysabri® treatments. After receiving Tysabri®, a very small number of patients had been diagnosed with a rare and potentially fatal brain infection called *progressive multifocal leukoencephalopathy* (PML). As a result of these concerns, Tysabri® was withdrawn from the market in 2005.

After extensive testing, it returned to the market in 2006 with a very detailed safety protocol to monitor patients for any PML concerns. As of December of 2010 the total number of confirmed cases of PML was 79, with 16 deaths (Reuters, December 2010).

It has been important for me to keep this statistic in perspective, because over 75,000 patients have used Tysabri® since its introduction. It was also noted that the rate of PML increases with the length of time that a person is on the drug—specifically, after 2 years. While Biogen Idec reports that the rate of PML is still within the 1-in-1,000 level, similar to the clinical trials and as cited on the label, they have actively pursued a method to identify and predict PML risk factors for patients receiving Tysabri®. At the time of this writing, researchers were developing a test for antibodies to the JC virus, which might help clinicians work out which patients on the drug could be at risk of developing PML.

While some would suggest that the numbers of people who had a fatal case of PML were statistically small, compared with the large number of those who have received Tysabri®, this was a sobering concern and obviously taken seriously by Biogen Idec when it removed the drug from the U.S. market. Given Tysabri®'s highly effective results for MS patients, individuals have to weigh for themselves whether developing the rare PML was worth the risk. When Tysabri® was reintroduced, Biogen Idec and FDA regulators agreed that those who use it would be closely monitored, along with timely reporting of any additional PML cases.

This is a composite of what I read from readily available news sources and additional information that was published by Biogen Idec. It not only made sense to me, but the PML safety concerns seemed well monitored and may soon be predictable. Anyone who is considering starting any approved medication for MS is strongly encouraged to gather all current information and consult with their medical provider and support person or team. These decisions may alter the course of MS differently for each person. A thoroughly informed decision to select a particular treatment should be made on an individual basis and not based upon rumor or false alarm.

My first-line therapy, Avonex®, was a very successful experience. After the short use of Rebif® and continued appearance of new lesions,

Dr. Thomas felt that Tysabri® was an appropriate consideration. Whether Tysabri® may be more useful as a first-line therapy or is used only after other therapies have been unsuccessful is a decision for each person with MS, after consultation with their medical provider. No hard and fast rule seems to apply to all. All of these concerns were part of my decision and should be independently weighed by each MS individual. If there ever was a time for me to gather trusted opinions on moving forward with Tysabri®, this was that moment.

"Do you think that PML is something that could affect you?" asked Terri. She had finished reading all the disclosure materials regarding Tysabri® that I had received from Biogen Idec. "I don't recall hearing about anyone dying with any of the other medications." She had nailed the question on the head. "How common is that?"

"No one is hiding that question and it was the first thing that grabbed my attention," I answered. "From what I have studied, a little more than a dozen MS patients have died from PML, since it was launched in 2004." After talking to Dr. Thomas, I felt more confident that my medication history did not put me at any risk or present any similarity to those who had developed PML. I had no interest in overlapping any other MS medication with Tysabri®. Dr. Thomas and I were on this same page.

"It is important that you read everything about the TOUCH program," said Dr. Thomas, "and ask me any questions if you have any concerns. I have a number of other patients on Tysabri® and we follow the program very closely. You should count on spending at least 2 hours here for the infusion. While the forms, questions, and actual infusion may only take an hour," he continued, "we like to keep an eye on you for another hour afterwards. If there would be any reaction at all, then we can catch it while you are sitting in the infusion room."

I was introduced to Marilyn, a comforting infusion nurse who was responsible for the detailed Tysabri® procedure. She would ensure that each patient was authorized to receive every Tysabri® infusion and confirm that the medication guide was read, verbally understood, and documented—each time. Although the infusion could become routine, strict adherence to completing the Patient Checklist and complying with the TOUCH program was serious and confidence building.

Being well informed about your MS therapy may help to ensure that you are following the recommended safety protocol.

The MS TOUCH Prescribing Program is detailed and leaves no relevant bit of MS patient information untouched. It felt like the monitoring rivaled the government's protocol for moving nuclear fuel across the country, but it provided a strong safety net of support to catch any sign of a problem. During an appointment with Dr. Matthais to discuss Tysabri®, she seemed to watch my eyes, perhaps looking for any sign of hesitation to start the therapy and then she took the conversation in a different direction.

"You have been on Avonex® for a long time," said Dr. Matthais, "do you have any concerns about having an infusion?"

"This may seem odd," I answered, "but I think that I would prefer an IV." Dr. Matthais put down her pen on a pad of paper. "For the first time, I wouldn't have to prepare the medication, syringe or inject myself. I may drink a lot of juice prior and then have to sit there for a couple of hours, but the injection part takes three seconds and the needle is gone." The infusion line that is left inserted into my vein remains painlessly taped up to my arm. "Removing the tape and pulling off some hair on my arm will probably be the most painful part of the process."

"Can you shave that area on your arm?" asked Dr. Matthais, suggesting the direct and practical approach. I nodded my head, picturing a bare surface on my arm for the infusion and tape. Despite being surrounded by shelves filled with medical books and articles, Dr. Matthais avoided distractions when sharing her insights. All of these mind-filling items, plus the computer screen and keyboard, were behind her and away from an easy gaze. Her desk was always so clear of distractions that I figured it was a key to maintaining focus on the conversation. All she could see was the person in the other chair, a clean desk top, and hear conversation between them. That nondistracting atmosphere allowed me to focus on each personal topic. This time, it provided a clear view to answer any lingering Tysabri® questions. It was all on the table.

"I spoke with Dr. Thomas and he mentioned that you could wait a month after stopping Rebif®, before your first Tysabri® infusion."

"Even when you stop," I said, "I guess the medication stays in the system for quite a while, maybe 30 days, so it is good to let it wash out before starting a different therapy. The exacerbation risk during in-between weeks seems low." My layperson description may not have medically impressed Dr. Matthais, but she seemed to generally agree with the concept. If I had misunderstood my condition or the use of Tysabri®, I knew that either Dr. Thomas or Dr. Matthais would have said something. Although I had separate conversations with each member of my MS "Team," it seemed like a single conversation with everyone in the room.

From their different perspectives, educational backgrounds, and qualifications, we all seemed to have gleaned the same information and conclusions regarding Tysabri®. It was clearly a powerfully effective MS therapy and as long as all of the proper methods and tests for monitoring my progress were followed, I did not have any real concern for myself about PML. None. With Terri's support, it was left as my call, with the decks cleared of second guessing. I would not look over my shoulder during the infusion, because I was surrounded by those who were supporting me in the game.

After weighing any potential risks for myself, I decided that I had a more realistic risk of getting into a car accident on the way to the infusion, rather than suffering any problem with the therapy and I decided that doing nothing was still not an option. For me, Tysabri® would be a great therapy to help maintain the essential pieces of my life, while waiting for the next better therapy or maybe a cure.

"Don't know how reliable this is, but my gut tells me that I will be fine with Tysabri®," I said to Terri.

"It helps to know that your doctors see Tysabri® the same way and support the choice," said Terri. This decision isn't like walking along the edge of a cliff in the dark. After discussing it with Terri and Drs. Thomas and Matthais, I felt confident that I had an informed decision at hand and was prepared to change therapy tracks and go forward. Terri and I finished our evening coffee and stood up from the kitchen table. We enjoyed one of the best long hugs that I can remember.

Even while considering another change in my MS treatment, I was mindful to continue managing my ongoing MS symptoms. The time in between medications would be no different. During the pause in between therapies, my body and mind continued to be weighed down by fatigue, slowing my movement and thoughts. Short naps do help me to regain a little focus and energy and on some days, two naps are needed to get to the dinner hour—and be sitting up and alert. There are no commercial breaks from MS. My PT and OT exercises, as well as engaging my mind in reading books, cognitive-based computer puzzles, writing, and volunteering MS advocacy never ceased. Waiting for my first Tysabri® infusion to begin, I would not leave a door open for MS.

> While compiling information about medication therapies, give no more ground to MS.

One of two immediate benefits to starting the Tysabri® regimen was that a therapy procedure was removed from our home, along with all of the needles, medication, and the smell of alcohol wipes. The Tysabri® infusions by a nurse were scheduled for every 28 days in a clinic. There was nothing for me to order, store, measure, inject, or properly dispose of into a red Sharps container. Terri didn't have to inject me, and our girls would never have to ask about the red box carefully stowed in the kitchen closet.

The other benefit was the loss of something. For me, Tysabri® held *none* of the flu-like side effects that I had experienced with Avonex® and tripled with Rebif®. With Tysabri®, I experience an occasional lingering dull headache, but that is manageable without seriously adding to my MS disability. There would be no additional fatigue burden placed on top of the MS fatigue and the hours and day(s) after the infusion were left as just another MS day. It may be unnoticeable to others, but it is a beautiful gift to me and others using Tysabri®.

> Each MS therapy may present different side effects for each person.

The infusion nurse, Marilyn, would handle the first treatment, preceded by the TOUCH program questions. She took an initial blood pressure measurement from me and prepared the Tysabri® drip bag, syringe, and lines for the infusion.

"And here is the poke," said Marilyn. She confidently hit the vein with one slight jab and immediately removed the needle, leaving only the IV infusion line. I glanced up to see the methodical drops of Tysabri® silently flow into my vein. Through my earphones, Norah Jones was already singing, "Come Away With Me," and my mind agreed to leave the room.

"That's as good as an injection gets," I said. "It is probably all in my mind, but I like the Butterfly needles, even if they are the same gauge as the others. Can we stay with those until I become afraid of butterflies?"

"It also seems to be much easier if you have a lot of liquids before the infusion," said Marilyn, "easier to hit the right spot the first time." As a patient, I couldn't agree more. "I need to get your blood pressure one more time before I get you more cranberry juice, and then I will let you go back into your music zone." Marilyn could watch me through the glass window by her computer and she would frequently check on me until I was out of the clinic. Her care was tender and thorough. After several months of infusions the TOUCH program questions became familiar, yet Marilyn never skipped a beat or lost sight of their benchmark purpose. I wasn't in this by myself.

"At your next infusion," said Judy, Dr. Thomas's medical assistant, "we should also get an antibody blood test from you and we may as well schedule your next MRI."

"Can we do it all at once, on the same day?" I asked.

"Sure and if we schedule it right," continued Judy, "then you will only need the one infusion poke. We can use the same line to draw a blood sample and then cap it until they need to insert the contrast agent during the MRI."

"If you can set that up for me to go right from the infusion into the MRI without a separate injection," I said, "then I'm in."

"No problem, I'll set it all up while you are here for the second hour." Three procedures from one infusion poke. It was a brilliant idea and Judy is an angel.

"As long as we got you here for a while," said Judy, "would you mind signing some of your books for us? We received a shipment of about 70 copies of your first book for our MS patients and it would be great to hand out signed copies."

"As long as I can sign without moving the taped-down Tysabri® line in my arm," I answered, "then stack them up next to that hand." Judy brought the large cardboard box of books into the infusion room and placed it on the floor—thump. A woman was sitting in another reclining "infusion" chair and was receiving a steroid treatment. She watched as Judy piled the books near my infusion arm and helped me to slide the first book under my signing hand.

"If it's O.K.,"I said, "then I'll neatly just drop them back in the box as I sign them."

"Take your time and let me know if you have any difficulty doing this, I don't want to mess up the infusion." Judy's heart always showed a caring light. All 70 were signed without missing a Tysabri® drop. After about a year of infusions, I was in the clinic for one of my regular appointments with Dr. Thomas.

"You have had a dozen or so infusions," said Dr. Thomas. "How do you feel about the Tysabri® decision?"

"No regrets," I answered, "and I honestly believe that it is the best MS thing that has come my way, since being diagnosed back in '96."

"Have you noticed any improvements?" asked Dr. Thomas.

"Removing the medication side effects was huge," I answered, "and I have found a little more energy to cope with numbness, stumbling, and mentally losing myself. Maybe the brain lesions can't go away, but with Tysabri® I feel like I have stopped losing ground to MS." Less drained energy and the ability to better cope with MS is an improvement—definitely.

"There's a school of thought that at the two-year mark," continued Dr. Thomas, "a 'drug holiday' would be beneficial in relation to PML concerns."

"I have no concern for myself about a rare instance of PML and unless the 'drug holiday' involves a week down in Cozumel with my family," I said, "then I'm not interested. Do you feel that any concern is justified?"

"No, there are no studies to support the benefit of a 'drug holiday' and no guarantee that in the interim MS exacerbations wouldn't occur," answered Dr. Thomas. "It is understandable that some might think that this is a way to avoid any PML, but there is no real evidence of it."

> Consider staying on your MS therapy until otherwise recommended by your medical professional.

"Without a published study to back up the theory and if you are not seeing anything to give you pause, then I'm sticking with the program. Tysabri® is going fine, we thoroughly discussed the therapy and I am confident with the TOUCH program. So I am not messing with it."

"I agree with you," said Dr. Thomas, "but I wanted you to be aware of what is floating around out there. I think there is more potential harm by temporarily stopping Tysabri®."

"And until I see something different, I am staying the course," I said. MS doesn't take a vacation and I will not open the door and invite it to join me on a "holiday." No, thank you. For me, the benefits of Tysabri® far outweigh the unsubstantiated second guessing by others.

Tips for Living

- ◆ Discover where new treatments will take you and halt MS, blocking it from severing vital neurological connections. Just imagine that.
- ◆ You are not responsible for having MS. Nothing is predetermined in your care and coping with MS, so be open to purposeful changes to maintain your well-being. Nurture your resiliency to adapt. This is a legacy worthy of your strength.
- ◆ For myself, I strongly believe that all MS therapies exist as a bridge until the next better treatment is available. Since the time when the A-B-C therapies were considered new, the MS community has been inspired by newer promising therapies. It is a sign of hope for all of us.

◆ Be sure that your MS conversation is well informed and supported by your personal MS network and homework. Engage with physicians, therapists, and MS organizations that understand and answer your concerns. Otherwise, seek out a trusted referral for a reliable second opinion. Listen through reliable sources to those who have successfully been there and done that.

◆ Stay tuned to scientifically based MS research and results and be leery of unproven recommendations, especially those based upon an isolated testimony. Do your research and remember that another word for "anecdotal" is "unreliable." Judge for yourself.

◆ Take ownership of the information and procedures for your MS treatment and medication and move forward with confidence, based upon trusted opinions regarding your care.

CHAPTER FOURTEEN

Gathering New Pieces

Wellness

In non-Olympic years, the oval ice at the Pettit National Ice Center is melted down for the spring and summer months. So what do a retired speedskater and any person with MS do for the rest of the year to stay cool and in decent shape? Alright, swimming is wet fun, but I have never had the right body mass to be naturally buoyant and instead, quickly reach exhaustion fighting to keep my head above water. Clinging to the side of the pool, while trying to exercise and not bang my knees into the grainy wall, restricted my movements and brought curious stares from the lifeguards. People do swim in Wisconsin, but it doesn't come to me with natural ease.

Due to MS problems with balance and numbness, made far worse by overheating, I was forced to surrender my running shoes within a few years after my MS diagnosis. The red Nike swoosh sits in a corner of the closet waiting for a different life. Any physical strain that raises my core body temperature is problematic, leaving me with noodle limbs and a fogged mind. Even a brisk walk leads me to gazing to the nearby ground searching for a spot of *soft* cement to crash. This is an unwanted coping mechanism and any impact strengthening from hitting the ground is not effective or recommended. MS reminds me that I need make a habit of taking care of myself to avoid losing vitality to an unprepared mind and body.

When my body is fatigued and I don't have the energy to walk with my daughter, MS is my overheated body struggling to balance and move. MS is cruel.

When I have trouble filling out a check because the blanks suddenly don't make sense, MS is there cutting holes in my concentration.

When I need to grab the railing to safely go up the stairs, MS is the drop-foot stumble in my gait.

When MS knocks clear thoughts out of my head or my body to the ground, I must be prepared to meet the daily challenge with an equal effort to strengthen my wellness.

Decide that taking care of yourself is a priority.

Any preparation must occur well in advance of those moments when I especially need to rely on my body and mind. The effort should be realistic for my MS limitations, and it must be a comfortable fit for my day. No one can be hired to do this for me, nor is there a computer icon to click, that instantly improves my condition, but there is a personal method that I welcomed into my life to counter the intrusion of MS. For me, a mildly structured physical workout not only maintains my stamina and muscle tone, it directly sparks cognitive activities. The grueling reality is that every form of exercise, physical therapy, and cross-training requires a specific level of commitment. Without it, you will pay with less energy, ability, along with diminishing focus and interest.

When I would skip a couple of days or a week without any physical workout, I paid for it with increased fatigue and less concentration or awareness. I would look for an elevator, rather than take the short flight of stairs. The book that I was reading would be closed on the bookmark and left on the carpet near the leg of my reading chair. My bookmark, a blue aerial Tram ticket from Jackson Hole, would peek out from the pages as if calling, "Don't forget to come back." Whenever given a chance, MS would cut in on my life dance like an interloper—killing the moment.

Neither the hard-polished oval ice nor my local health club can travel with me and I searched to find consistency in my personal workout, avoiding easy excuses. Since MS is present in my life every day without exception, I needed to find movements to meet MS every day. Any benefit will not occur by itself; however, an opportunity to construct a reasonable fit for myself tapped me on the shoulder. There would be a free exercise DVD that would be made available to the MS community, just for asking. There would be three levels of exercises demonstrated for the viewers and I was asked to participate in one of the filmed groups demonstrating the MS Active Wellness program.

> One exercise program does not fit everyone; find the MS group that best matches your needs and abilities.

In an effort to provide a comfortable fitness path for each person with MS, there would be three separate exercise groups: a chair-based *Vitalize* workout, an *Energize* workout (my group) that used a chair for balance, and finally, a *Maximize* workout for a physically challenging workout routine. Each workout is about an hour long, but you can personalize the routine to fit your needs, timing, and abilities, incorporating weights where desired to build strength. No one is watching or judging you, but you can skip the rainbow-colored spandex.

Each workout is led by a fitness coach, Katrina Hodgson, who invites you to connect the desire for fitness to your overall wellness. The DVD is immediately engaging because of its easy-to-follow movements and interspersed casual conversations with the MS participants. The trilevel program was created with the guidance of Dr. Barry Hendin, a leading neurologist and authority on the management of MS. The simple and realistic goal of the DVD is to keep persons with MS moving and motivated with a program created for all levels of ability. The Wellness fitness program is a crucial link in managing the physical and cognitive challenges of MS. For each person with MS, the Wellness program advises that when a person with MS selects and follows a workout (with physician approval where appropriate), it may help them by

- *improving flexibility and decreasing muscle weakness and stiffness;*
- *reducing spasticity and other MS symptoms;*

♦ *increasing strength and decreasing likelihood of experiencing fatigue;*

♦ *improving mood and overall total body health/wellness.*

Without the commitment to move the body and energize the mind, each person with MS faces a one-sided battle with diminishing returns.

> **People with MS do not give up.**

The filming for the DVD was arranged in a Los Angeles film studio, and once each fitness group passed through rehearsal and then through the benefit of makeup and hair styling, we were prepared to exercise. For DVD viewers, the program reminds everyone to have water, a comfortable mat, and a wet towel at hand for the scheduled cool-down checkpoints, although breaking a sweat isn't a necessary part of each routine. However, the temperature in the L.A. studio rapidly climbed for us during filming, since the air-conditioning needed to be turned off to avoid recording its running sound. Our *Energize* group did not require an unusual number of retakes, but for those of us in our group who do not deal well with heat, the varying studio steam was unwelcome. The towels were great, and when I messed up the makeup to dab perspiration, the makeup lady was ready to touchup any shine.

The workout was honest and when I grabbed the chair to catch myself from falling, there was no edit cut. When I lost count of the number of repetitions, no edit cut. The individuals in each group have MS and their abilities and limitations are reflected by what they could comfortably accomplish or not—no edit cut. If you have MS, then you will probably be able to identify with someone from one of the groups, since none of us with MS can edit out our difficult moments. Interviews with each participant are also available on the DVD and Web site, sharing insights and their motivation, saying: "You can do it too." It is all MS-real and welcomes each person to join with one of the workout groups that works best for their fitness level.

"Engage your core," said Katrina as she spoke to our *Energize* group, "and I don't mean suck in your gut or hold your breath."

She approached me from the side and gently placed her hand in the middle of my back, between my shoulder blades, and explained that I should keep my shoulders back, as if trying to pinch her hand between the blades. When I focused on keeping my shoulders down, square, and a bit back, then the rest of my body seemed to align itself and was better balanced. My stomach muscles fell comfortably under my rib cage, probably where they belong. MS tends to make many folks, myself included, hunch over from fatigue, and sometimes favor one limb over another. My prior poor stance became obvious to me and now felt straightened out and natural.

"Remember to breathe and keep your shoulders back," said Katrina, "and think of leading your body with your chest and heart forward." Of course, she was speaking more figuratively and not emotionally.

Whether sitting or standing, poor MS posture throws everything else out of whack and creates other balance and movement difficulties. Save this spent energy for other demands in your life. My phrasing may not be the best fitness terminology, but if you can visualize my descriptions or better yet, request and watch a copy of the DVD, then you will see for yourself how easy it is to carry yourself in a manner that can make physical activity less stressful. All of the movements seem to start from this basic posture of engaging your "core." If you try this out, then you too may be able to exercise, stretch, and move with more grace and energy. When I do so, it also seems to fuel my cognitive awareness and makes things a little easier to notice and absorb. Merely watching the DVD offers no such benefits, so select a fitness group that is comfortable for you and start there.

> Find your core strength and let it be the basis of your wellness.

The difference felt in my life by embracing a flexible exercise routine was easy to notice. When I have skipped a few days and have not stretched my body or made much of an effort to maintain the strength of my core, everything takes more energy and feels out of sync. My body doesn't move as well as it should and my thoughts are rapidly jammed and memory exhausted. The Tin Man in *The Wizard of Oz* found it difficult to move or speak after not using his body and letting the rust stop all motion. If he had taken better care of himself by keeping his joints lubricated and avoided the rain or had an umbrella, then he would have been able to continue chopping trees. Instead, he rusted and wasn't able to move. Without any guided fitness movement, you may also find yourself unable to shake loose some rust.

The *Energize* group workout is my "oilcan" of smooth movement and I need to use it on a regular basis to avoid slowing down. The benefit is ripe to grasp like a morning stretch when you roll out of bed to begin your day. Without that first deep breath-yawn in the morning and an invigorating stretch of your arms and legs, firing a spark of energy and the blood flowing, you would probably tumble back onto the bed. Leaping out of bed with a cheerful disposition has never been automatic. I have to get myself moving and just not think about it.

On days when time is tight and I am deciding what items I can save for another day, it would be easy to ignore energizing my body. To save time, it would be easy enough to skip a meal, but my body would know that its sustenance was missing. I would crash, paying for the lack of sustaining nutrition. Even a light lunch of cinnamon raisin oatmeal or granola yogurt is better than nothing at all and keeps me moving. For fitness, an equally quick combination of leg lifts, ankle turns, and body positions like the plank are vitalizing. These *Energize* bites are my *fitness snacks* during each day and are not to be skipped. I can *snack* anywhere.

It was important for me to avoid excuses and doing nothing, so I adjusted the exercises, timing, and repetitions based upon the model on the DVD. There is no single locked way to complete a routine. My weekly schedule contains three full workouts and a lot of *fitness snacking* on the other days. For easy reference, I have a printed list of the *Energize* group exercises. Incorporating the exercises from our *Energize* group, this is my routine and I have committed to its purpose and benefits, while feeling the direct results.

To a greater or lesser extent, I run through the exercises practically every day and I can take the list with me on the road. MS may affect the amount of time that I feel able to dedicate to the workout, but it doesn't stop me from reaching for fitness to improve my wellness. It also has to be flexible, engaging, and work for you or it won't last for long. Following the DVD with my L.A. friends, I am definitely not alone and I am moving with newfound energy.

Whether fighting MS through complementary therapies or one of the approved medication treatments, don't stop actively pursuing your choice of fitness for physical and cognitive flexibility. Maybe we can't pick our MS symptoms, but you can select a level of discipline to maintain your wellness. Choose to follow the model of others who are resiliently living with MS. Do not surrender.

Staying Smart

Being connected to others living with MS may be the most underappreciated way to stay physically fit, remain on your MS therapy, and to be motivated to move your thoughts away from the grip of MS. Arranging these connections is a personal choice for each individual with MS, since the disease can batter each person in a different way. Five people may separately sit in the driver's seat of the same car, but they will each adjust the seat to fit their personal needs. Once settled behind the wheel, learning from others how to safely navigate the roads can save a person a lot of frustration and keep them from ending up in the wrong place.

At the time of my MS diagnosis, cognitive tour maps didn't exist and trip tickets were unavailable. For those people trying to recognize the signs of their own MS mental detours and hazards, they were alone to machete their own survival trail. Although more than half of the MS population has been dealing with some level of cognitive difficulties, there are few opportunities for those MS individuals to participate in ongoing discussions, sharing their confusion, as well as their practical tips and tools. An open and available exchange about enduring an MS cognitive life is overdue and would be welcomed.

> People dealing with MS cognitive challenges are not alone and definitely wish to help each other. Look for support groups or online boards if you are so inclined.

When I learned that there was going to be a cognitive Web site tool developed by the MS Trust U.K. specifically for people with MS and their health care professionals, it was an exciting moment and a dream come true. I was asked to be a member of the Expert Review Panel to look over the draft version of the site and provide feedback about the Web site. I joined the panel and privately celebrated when the cognition site www.stayingsmart.com.org.uk was launched. In 2009, I was asked to participate in a filmed discussion in London with other people dealing with the cognitive challenges of MS. The filmed comments from the participants may be found on the Web site for the MS Trust and probably YouTube. The MS Trust asked me to write an article about what was learned that day for publication in their magazine (*Open Door*). The article is reprinted here.

Staying Smart and Staying Afloat (*Open Door*, February 2010, pages 8–9)

By Jeffrey N. Gingold

To a casual observer it might appear that we are an ocean apart. When the MS Trust asked me to participate in a filmed group discussion, regarding the cognitive challenges of multiple sclerosis, the Atlantic distance between my home in the United States and London vanished. MS is not halted by a shoreline and neither are the efforts to cope with it.

In fact, those of us living with multiple sclerosis are sitting next to each other in the same boat, enduring stealth cognitive slams from MS lesions. Since at least half of the MS population is faced with thinking difficulties, there is no reason to remain silent on the turbulent ship. There are mental life jackets, but each person with MS needs to find the one that fits them. Discovering what keeps an MS mind well connected begins with acknowledging thinking difficulties and then learning successful coping tactics, often from others in the MS community. Were you told to handle MS setbacks by yourself? Probably not. Wouldn't you ask for directions in a foreign city and rely on those who know the way? There is nothing wrong with letting someone else drive, just like taking a taxi.

Arriving in London, I realised that my loss of presence in an MS cognitive moment is very much like experiencing a taxi ride in London. En route to the hotel for the MS Trust presentation, our driver noticed our American accents and asked if we enjoyed driving on the "other side" of the road. My daughters, Lauren and Meredith, were thrilled by the experience of the driver sitting on the right side of the vehicle and driving on the left side of the road—backwards to us.

I chose to not contemplate how I would safely operate a car in this mirrored existence and gladly accepted the assistance of the driver to navigate the streets. To the gleeful squeals of our girls, the driver stated "but you prefer to drive over here, don't you?" He playfully careened the taxi into the right lane and zoomed toward the on-coming cars. Just short of sending the terrified traffic onto the sidewalk, he cut back to the left lane. My cognitive moments are like that, suddenly forgetting what I am doing or losing my place in a conversation or location, finding myself on the "other side" of the road and unsure what to do next.

On that warm, blue sky day in June, they came from across the country and battled trains and Tubes to share their MS cognitive experiences. The MS Trust had recently launched its cutting-edge StayingSmart website as an open invitation for the MS community to "learn, build and share" a better cognitive understanding. This interactive site would assemble the best techniques to handle the MS cognitive challenges that are privately experienced by people with MS.

Make no mistake about it—there is an invisible stigma about cognitive challenges. It is difficult for people to move out of their initial denial phase when they are not educated about that part of MS and their doctor won't go there. If that discussion never starts, then the patient is caught in a circle of denial, leading to more denial. As I sat down for the presentation with a microphone clipped inside my shirt collar, the cameras began to roll and I wondered whether the attendees would run silent and slip into that denial. When asked whether anyone had any tips or tricks to share, the outpouring of personal cognitive skills began to flow. Collectively, they kicked open the door of MS cognitive discussion.

"Lists are very good, lists and lists and lists," said a woman, as she emphasised keeping track of thoughts, as well as remembering where the lists are placed for future reference.

Another woman stated that when cognitive problems began for her, she was unsure whether it was simply related to her fatigue.

"When I was diagnosed," said another lady, "I had a very stressful job where I had to spin a lot of plates." It had become commonplace for her to lose the thread of a thought, leaving her with "a horrible, sinking feeling."

Even though I was thousands of miles from home, the conversation mirrored the MS community in my neighbourhood. Those who are coming to grips with mental impediments are surprised to learn that they are not alone in their word finding difficulties, loss of concentration, mental fatigue and other untimely cognitive symptoms. Actually, it is a crowded room.

"You think that you're just imagining it all," stated another man with MS. The concerns were real and the level of honesty was astounding. He noted that "to lose being a 'thinker' can be the scariest thing about MS." Heads in the room began to nod in strong agreement. Others discussed the loss of short-term memory and the methods for delegating tasks to other people, whether at home or work. More head nods.

Wanting to keep those bewildering cognitive moments to yourself tends to make matters worse, especially when others can't see the mental shutdown. Whether the word is caught on the tip of your tongue, conversations are confounded or you lost a train of thought, others may not understand the cognitive derailment. The jammed process is invisible, except for the frustration registered on your face. When it is taking you more time to accomplish less at work or on home projects, simply because you feel overwhelmed by multi-task details that were once manageable, this is also your MS, but you are not alone. Many of us dealing with MS have been there too.

A lady stated how her husband is far more patient now that he understands why she suddenly changes subjects in the middle of a conversation without even being aware of it. By sharing her experiences with MS cognitive misdirection, their relationship avoids collateral damage.

There is a new safe harbour to address your concerns, which will place the maps and tools in your hands to better navigate the cognitive turmoil of MS. When you look into your private soul, discover that you are at your best when you share and help another. That is the purpose and appeal of this website, since it is designed to help any person with MS to get their thoughts back on track. In this vast and confounding ocean, the steady boat is the MS Trust and the calm port is its new StayingSmart website for cognitive discussion. Know that whatever cognitive problem that you may face, there may already be an answer addressed by others who have already landed there.

That day in London, many individuals from the MS community reached out with an honest discussion. Their personal coping strategies are all there on the site and the video clips are easily accessible to the MS community at large. They are brave to open their private stories and share their mental sharpening techniques, so that others dealing with MS might benefit from the on-point direction—hold fast to a vital life with your families and friends.

Whether in MS high seas, calm rivers or running against the tide, check out the cognitive sharing in your midst and begin to enjoy the benefits of sitting next to each other—smooth sailing and stay smart.

The MS Trust has created and tipped over a large domino, pushing forward the discussion of MS cognitive concerns and coping techniques. The ripple effects are spreading like a record-breaking dominos demonstration. Click onto this sharing discussion—no passport is necessary to stay smart.

A Way Through

"What are you using?" asked a woman who abruptly cornered me after my presentation at an MS cognition seminar. "How do you function with MS?" She pushed herself toward me, blocking my path to the book-signing table. Over her shoulder I could see people politely waiting in line.

"Happy to answer your question," I answered, "but maybe we could talk in more detail after the signing." She folded her arms and then shifted her stance to not let me pass by.

"What do you take for your MS!?" she continued. "I am also an ER nurse, so you can tell me." Her question had an insistent urgency to it, like that of a scuba diver low on air and 100 feet underwater. Deciding to receive a well-documented MS treatment (Tysabri®) and pursuing wellness was a process with a personal commitment. It is not a quick or easy answer for any person with MS.

During the past several years, MS cognitive presentations have provided me with opportunities to share what I have experienced, but not to suggest that there is a universal solution that provides a perfectly normal life with MS. I am not sure that one exists and I certainly don't possess it. A person may firmly demand an Olympic Gold Medal, but there is no switch or pill for instantly placing them in front of the Olympic finish line. It also doesn't exist.

My MS path is imperfect with some wrong turns and it continues to be a work in process, until there is a cure. Although there are no magic shoes to transport a person into a better condition, just know that the therapies and techniques exist to improve a life with MS. These are my primary tools against MS and I share them to encourage others to stay physically strong and cognitively sharp, plus find time to give extra hugs.

Tips for Living

- Learn about your body with MS and how to promote its mental and physical strength.
- Engage and control your personal wellness. No amount of written material, medication, and supplements can substitute for safely moving your body and stimulating your mind.
- Make your fitness routine be fun and easy to access. Use the proven experience of others to inspire your best health, but not as a substitute for self-action.
- Whether connected with MS information online, through conferences, or one-on-one discussions, don't hesitate to learn from others who have successfully adapted to their MS impediments.
- Have confidence in your resilience and the spirit that guides it. MS may only remit if we continue to surrender no ground and give no quarter to its symptoms. Fight back with all of the resources at your disposal and take care of yourself by staying engaged in your conditioning and treatment.
- Be your own game-changer.

In Summation . . .

"Can I help you find something?" asked the teenage boy, as he walked toward me along the wooded path. My walking pace had been slowed by fatigue, and the distance between us had lessened. But it wasn't a concern about my toes clearing the ground that was slowing me down. He thought I was lost because I appeared to be confused by my surroundings.

"No," I said, "I just need to rest for a few minutes." He smiled, spun around, and ran back toward the main lodge. Of course, I have been both individuals in this scene, but being disabled by the cognitive re-routing of multiple sclerosis does not mean that I am unable to reach out to others with the disease. Part of me is still that Hollar Park camp counselor I was so long ago, only now I am helping others move themselves along the invisible, jagged path of MS disability. Assisting the National Multiple Sclerosis Society offers me the pleasure of meeting the varied faces of MS and sharing common difficulties with others, despite having my mental and physical legs often knocked out from under me.

The people I speak to every day in my capacity as a volunteer are nothing short of amazing. They are heroes who deserve an award for rising each morning and traversing the day with whatever challenges MS puts before them. Everyone has a story about facing the grinding pressures of a job, finances, and family, but people with MS do all that while carrying the burden of a disabling disease. They get through it somehow, and then they welcome another day. They are the courageous ones who have survived the shock and denial of an MS diagnosis—a disease that, so far, has no cure. The goal for each of them is to find their own pathway to resolution and action, and then find the determination to follow that path.

People who have had their lives pummeled by multiple sclerosis, shaken to the core of their very humanity, will never know why they have been afflicted by such a relentless and devastating disease. They don't deserve disability—period. What they do deserve is a *thorough* diagnosis of their multiple sclerosis and appropriate treatment and therapies. Given the opportunity to learn about the "thinking" side of multiple sclerosis and the measures that can be taken to stave off and cope with mental exacerbations, MS patients can better manage their lives. They have a remarkable ability to rise up and face the challenge, no matter how daunting the task may seem at first. Just like skaters who are surprised by suddenly falling, they know better than to just sit on the cold ice and wait. They pick themselves up, sometimes with the help of a family member or friend, and keep moving as best they can on the slippery ground.

Yet, despite the best intentions, multiple sclerosis and misinformation about the potency of its cognitive symptoms can get the best of a person. Having MS should never be about looking over your shoulder, just waiting for the next exacerbation. By moving forward with my life, I decided to not remain idle, trapped like a hunted animal. For each person with multiple sclerosis, there are genuine and substantive steps they can take against this relentless disease. If I can take the strides, despite the unreliability of cognition and limbs, then others can do it, too.

Goal Number One: Cognitive Education

No one is a helpless victim of MS, unless they allow themselves to be. Diminishing energy is better spent on looking forward, instead of dwelling on what may be lost. Your spirit can stand up to this mind- and body-distorting disease.

> A person with multiple sclerosis is more than just a person with a disability.

Self-education for the cognitive challenges of MS is partly about assembling a support team. Treatment by a neurologist who has a significant number of MS patients and understands the multifaceted aspects of the disease is crucial. Don't be afraid to ask questions about the doctor's experience and understanding of the disease. An informed neuropsychologist and other supporting therapists can define the cognitive impairments of MS and outline methods of coping, but only if the patient is first willing to open up and speak honestly about difficulties with recall, reasoning, or moments of mental confusion. Therapies and coping techniques are the most useful when they are clearly communicated to both the patient and the family members, who can be supportive in their application in daily life. *Remember Chapter Eight, when everyone at my house agreed how to put things away—scissors or extra keys included?*

Humor is a potent medicine and, quite often, it is the sanest way out of a befuddled incident. Laughing out loud at my mental lapses has saved me from melting down into tears or lashing out in anger on many occasions. Sometimes, it is nothing more than looking at your life as if you are living a segment of *America's Funniest Home Videos.* Allow yourself to take a "mental time-out" in order to gather your thoughts, and then calmly finish a conversation or activity.

Multiple sclerosis may disrupt your schedule and sentences, but with time and patience, you will find a way to get back on track. It doesn't matter whether you see the glass as being half empty or half full. Either way, you will take in the same amount, only slower and through a narrower straw. Just make sure that the straw is kept in the same kitchen drawer, and not left in different locations!

Goal Number Two: Take Action

Once you recognize and have evaluated the cognitive impact of MS on your life and career, significant changes in your life may be necessary. Where are you going to land, financially and emotionally, if your health is better off in retirement? You can begin to lay the groundwork for a transitional path by working with your doctors to find appropriate methods and activities to keep your mind active and sharp.

If you are feeling sorry for yourself, then make it quick and get over it. When you don't feel motivated, try volunteering to help others. Except in rare instances, multiple sclerosis is not a fatal diagnosis, like some other chronic diseases. People with ALS, Alzheimer's, or

AIDS are engaged in a fight for their lives. Thankfully, there are some answers for MS, and it can be battled openly. By taking care of myself and educating others about MS, I have hope for a near future *without* multiple sclerosis.

Remain active and live larger than before the MS. Allow any confusing cognitive moments that you experience as they are *only temporary*. Delay and confusion is *nothing,* unless you let it become *everything*. Don't be afraid to slow down and allow disorientation to dissipate. Your children, spouse, parents, and friends can be a source of strength and purpose, no matter what your situation entails. Find joy in subtle pleasures, such as the no-rush coloring with a child or relaxing in a garden, when you are compelled to slow down. Whether it's a ride in a hot air balloon or talking with a neighbor about spring plantings, be aware that you are alive and vital. Live vibrantly in the quiet concert of life.

Find joy in subtle pleasures and live vibrantly. After the most distracting and stressful burdens have been minimized, fill your mental space with political, artistic, religious, and family activities of personal passion. No doubt, the local chapter of the National Multiple Sclerosis Society would welcome your insights and involvement.

Each day provides constructive alternatives that utilize different abilities and provide a sense of purpose and accomplishment. As you strive for sharpness of mind and reliable fluidity of thought, remember that the need for rest is beneficial for the mind. It is also a reality of multiple sclerosis.

Simplify and compartmentalize the details and physical items in your life. You may not remember the information when you need it, but at least you will know where to find it—like Einstein.

Goal Number Three: Reach for Available Answers

Study the available research. You may already know about the fatigue and numbness associated with MS, but it is worthwhile to also become educated about the possible mental changes. The National Multiple Sclerosis Society offers a vast support network of seminars and written materials.

Millions of people have endured the disabling affects of multiple sclerosis, and have learned how to live productive lives. Knowledgeable doctors and therapists, along with the education and outreach of the NMSS, can provide the necessary tools for each MS patient to create their personal program for moving along with MS. With the proper diagnosis of cognitive symptoms and the promise of available medications, there is no reason for anyone with MS to silently flounder.

Family members deserve honest communication. Let them know how and when you need their help. They will assist you in removing obstacles if you give them the chance. Perhaps above all else, be especially diligent in caring for yourself.

"You look at peace," said Patrick, a friend who had not seen me since I retired. "I've never seen you look so relaxed."

I didn't have the heart to tell him the complicated truth. The peaceful appearance is not due to having MS, but the result of learning to deal with it as a part of my life. *The best moments are when I forget that I have multiple sclerosis. An even better moment is when I realize that despite MS, I am doing more than just surviving, I am truly living.*

Goal Number Four: Leave Room for Slow Hugs

Hold close the people you love. Be patient with them and with yourself. Remain determined to cherish and evolve your life, in spite of multiple sclerosis. Soon enough, your difficulties may be looked upon as being just another temporary thing in your past. Take care of yourself by remaining physically active and mentally sharp, buying time until a medication is developed that will further slow the disabilities of multiple sclerosis and, ultimately, produce a cure.

Living with the cognitive challenges of multiple sclerosis is not about being abandoned on the road. It is beyond merely surviving. Decide to seek a better understanding of your body's needs, a better quality of life, and a better appreciation of what is possible. By insisting on moving forward, realize that you still possess far more of your good life than what may have been lost. Find new directions that will take you where you need to go. Pursue and enjoy life, despite multiple sclerosis!

Resources

The articles, brochures, books, and contacts listed below can assist you in obtaining a better and more complete understanding of MS. Life with MS should be an informed existence, seasoned with humor and dignity. Learn all you can about how to take better care of yourself.

Articles and Brochures

J. Benito-Leon, J.M. Morales, and J. Rivera-Navarro. Health-related quality of life and its relationship to cognitive and emotional functioning in multiple sclerosis patients. *European Journal of Neurology,* September, 2002.

Julie A. Bobholz and Stephen M. Rao. Cognitive dysfunction in multiple sclerosis: A review of recent developments. *Current Opinion in Neurology.* 2004; 16(3): 283–288.

D. Buljevac, W.C. Hop, and W. Reedeker, et. al. Self-reported stressful life events and exacerbations in multiple sclerosis: a prospective study. *British Medical Journal,* September 2003; 327(7416):646.

Douglas R. Denney, Sharon G. Lynch, Brett A. Parmenter, et al. Cognitive impairment in relapsing and primary progressive multiple sclerosis: Mostly a matter of speed. *Journal of the International Neuropsychological Society,* November 2004; Vol.10; 07:948–956.

Paul J. Donoghue, Mary E. Siegel, and Gary Sumner, et al. On disclosing your MS. *National Multiple Sclerosis Society,* 1997.

Frederick Foley and Jane Sarnoff. Taming stress in multiple sclerosis. *National Multiple Sclerosis Society,* 2001.

INS: Multiple Sclerosis Patients with Cognitive Impairment Have Trouble Processing Information; http://www.pslgroup.com/dg/214B9E.htm; *Doctor's Guide,* February, 2002.

Nicholas LaRocca and Martha King, Solving Cognitive Problems, *National Multiple Sclerosis Society,* 2007.

Jean Lengenfelder. Multiple sclerosis patients with cognitive impairment have trouble processing. *International Neuropsychological Society*, February, 2002.

D.D. Mohr, D.E. Goodkin, and S. Nelson, et al. Moderating effects of coping on the relationship between stress and the development of new brain lesions in multiple sclerosis. *Psychosomatic Medicine* 2002; 64: 810–816.

Barry S. Oken. Yoga may combat MS fatigue, study presented at American Academy of Neurology's 55th Annual Meeting. Oregon Health and Science University (OHSU); 2003.

D.M. Pizzi. MS and cognition, real living with multiple sclerosis. 2003; www.avonex.com (found under "News and Research.").

Stephen M. Rao. Cognitive function in patients with multiple sclerosis: Impairment and treatment. *International Journal of MS Care*, 2004.

Allen E. Thornton, Naftali Raz, Karen A. Tucker. Memory in multiple sclerosis: Contextual encoding deficits. *Journal of the International Neuropsychological Society*, March 2002; Vol. 8; 3:395–409.

Cognitive Functioning, *A Clinical Bulletin from the Professional Resource Center of the National Multiple Sclerosis Society*, 2008.

Emotions and cognition: MS in focus. *Multiple Sclerosis International Federation*, Issue 4, 2004.

Informs New Outcomes Study Reports Tysabri, *International Journal of MS Care*, April 29, 2009.

MS and the mind, *Inside MS*, Spring, 2000.

MS Patients with Cognitive Impairment. *International Neuropsychological Society*, February, 2002.

Solving Cognitive Problems: Managing Specific Issues, N. LaRocca, & M. King, National Multiple Sclerosis Society, 2007.

Stress worsens multiple sclerosis, *British Medical Journal*, Fall 2003.

Treatment of Multiple Sclerosis: Related Cognitive Problems with Adjunctive Modafinil, Wilken, J.A., Sullivan C., Mitchell, W., et al., 2008.

Suggested Books

Climbing Higher, by Montel Williams, New American Library, 2004.

Blindsided: Lifting a Life Above Illness, by Richard M. Cohen, HarperCollins Publishers, 2004.

Strong at the Broken Places: Voices of Illness, a Chorus of Hope, by Richard M. Cohen, Harper, 2008.

Yoga and Multiple Sclerosis: A Journey to Health and Healing, by Loren Martin Fishman, B. Phil, Eric Small, Demos Medical Publishing, 2007.

Exercises for Multiple Sclerosis: A Safe and Effective Program to Fight Fatigue, Build Strength, and Improve Balance (Exercises for), by Brad Hamler, Hatherleigh, 2006.

Mental Sharpening Stones: Manage the Cognitive Challenges of Multiple Sclerosis, by Jeffrey N. Gingold, Demos Medical Publishing, 2008.

Multiple Sclerosis: Understanding the Cognitive Challenges, by Nicholas LaRocca & Rosalind C. Kalb, Demos Health, 2006.

The Multiple Sclerosis Manifesto: Action to Take, Principles to Live By, by Julie Stachowiak, Demos Health, 2010.

What Nurses Know, Multiple Sclerosis: The Answers You Need From the People You Trust, by Carol Saunders, Demos Medical Publishing, 2011.

Useful Contacts

Can Do Multiple Sclerosis, www.mscando.org
Consortium of Multiple Sclerosis Centers, www.mscare.org
International Organization of MS Nurses, www.iomsn.org
Multiple Sclerosis International Federation, www.msif.org
Multiple Sclerosis Foundation, www.msfocus.org
Montel Williams MS Foundation, www.montelms.org
MS World, www.msworld.org
Rocky Mountain MS Center, www.MSCenter.org
MS Society U.K., www.mssociety.org.uk
Multiple Sclerosis Resource Centre, www.msrc.co.uk
Multiple Sclerosis Society of Canada (Société canadienne de la sclérose en plaques), www.mssociety.ca
Consortium of Multiple Sclerosis Centers, www.mscare.org
National Multiple Sclerosis Society, www.nmss.org
MS ActiveSource, www.msactivesource.com
MS Trust, www.mstrust.org.uk
MS Trust StayingSmart, www.stayingsmart.org.uk

Patient Information

Almost all of the pharmaceutical companies that manufacture medications for the treatment of multiple sclerosis have financial support programs. Please contact the manufacturer directly or check with the

Web sites below for additional information about financial assistance.
Financial assistance may be available to you, if you ask.

www.needymeds.com

www.phrma.org

www.themedicineprogram.com

Index

acceptance of MS, 51, 54

Active Wellness program, 183

air conditioning to allay symptoms, 36, 39. *See also* heat and MS symptoms

Alzheimer's vs. MS, 47, 61, 141

anger management, 19, 23, 58, 66, 110, 139

Aricept®, 141

assistive devices, 95

Avonex®, 28, 70, 72–75, 78, 79, 97, 110, 113, 165–168, 170, 171. *See also* medications for MS

mentor programs for, 110

Barry, Hendin, Dr., 183

Baughn, Diane, 107

Bernie Mac, 93–95

Betaseron®, 28, 70. *See also* medications for MS

Biogen, 78. *See also* Avonex®; medications for MS

study, 170

Biogen Idec reports, 170, 171

blood testing, 33–35

brain lesions, 85, 86, 93, 126, 127, 167, 169, 177

Charcot, Jean-Martin, xvii

chronic disease, living with, 32, 82, 86, 197

cognitive difficulties in MS, 29–30, 42–43

Aricept® for, 141

incidence of, 61, 63, 110–112, 143

information overload and, 139

neuropsychological testing for, 44–47

organizing living/work space for, 102

others' experiences of, 143–144

recordkeeping for, 128

statistics on, xv

cognitive education, 196–197

communication, honest, 125

communication overload, dealing with, 39

back-up systems for, 128

cell phones, use for, 128

e-mail, as communication device in, 39

confusion

avoiding, 142

recording moments of mental, 128

Copaxone®, 28, 70. *See also* medications for MS

death from MS, 144

denial, 19, 23, 25, 29, 30

differential diagnosis for MS symptoms (other diseases mimicking MS), 18

disability, 4, 6, 8
  challenges faced by, 1–9
  discrimination against,
    1–9, 149
  insurance, 83–84
disorientation, 118
distinctive symptom management
  program, 108
driving and MS symptoms, 117–123
drug trials for MS, 33

e-mail, as communication
  device, 39
Easter Seals summer camp, 2
EEG test, 123, 124, 127
Einstein, Albert, 100
empowerment, 74
exercise groups, 183

Facilitator Flash, 148
family mask, 67–84
fatigue, 13–15, 29, 32, 36
  mental, 32
  physical, 32
  tips for preventing/dealing
    with, 65
First-line therapy, 172
fitness groups, 185
Flu-like symptoms, 73, 78, 165,
  168, 169, 175
Froedtert Memorial Lutheran
  Hospital, 44
funding for MS research, 146–150

gender in MS, 27

heat and MS symptoms, 10,
  13–17, 36
Hodgson, Katrina, 183
Hollar Park Easter Seals Camp, 8

home and office adaptations, 39
hugs, slow, importance of, 199

information overload, dealing
  with, 139
injectable medication, 28, 71.
  See also medications for MS
  learning to self inject, 72
InsideMS, 43, 112, 139
Interferon beta 1a, 165
*International Journal of MS
  Care,* 170
intravenous medication, 42

JC virus, 171

Kalt, Colleen, 149

Landers, David, 105–106
learning about MS, 144–145, 196
legislation and funding for MS
  research, 146–150
lesions, brain, 85, 86, 93, 126, 127,
  167, 169, 177
lesions of MS, 22, 55–56
  location of, vs. symptoms, 41–42
light and eye discomfort. *See* optic
  neuritis; vision problems
limping, 3
living/working space
  adapting your, 39
  organizing, 102
"loss of presence" feeling, xviii,
  53, 120

magnetic resonance imaging (MRI),
  19, 22, 33, 34, 41, 55, 166, 168
  contrast injections for, 21
  lesions of MS on, 22, 41–42,
    55–56

mask
　family, 67–84
　removing, 83
Matthais, Josie, 44
medications for MS, 27–29, 43,
　73, 169
　advertising for, 28
　Alzheimer's disease and, 141
　choice of, 64
　decision to begin, 43, 51
　drug trials to develop, 33
　empowerment through, 74
　injectable, 28, 71
　intravenous, 42
　learning to self inject, 72
　manufacturers of, 82, 110
　mentor programs for, 110
　MS-fighting, 70
　oral, 34
　reviewing options for, 64–65
　self-injecting, 79
　side effects of, 42, 73–74,
　　78–79
　slowing of MS progression
　　through use of, 69
　steroid, 75
　symptom management to, 27
memory problems, 52–53,
　61, 100
　Aricept for, 141
　devices to aid, 101
　not recognizing significant
　　people and places in, 129–137
　organizing living/work space
　　for, 102
mental confusion, recording
　moments of, 128
mental disorientation of MS,
　100, 118
mental lapses of MS, 120, 130

mental wheelchair, drifting and
　dragging in, 129–142
mentor programs, 110
Milwaukee Public Museum, 104
misinformation about MS,
　144–145
MRI. *See* magnetic resonance
　imaging
MS Connections, 106, 147
MS-fighting medication, 70
MS Trust, 188–192
MS-Walk, 148
multiple sclerosis (MS)
　acknowledging, cognitive
　　challenges, 65–66
　cognitive impact of, 197
　diagnosis of, 25, 29, 146, xvii
　differential diagnosis for, 18
　disclosure of, 29
　exacerbation, 99, 120, 121
　intrusion of, 182
　mental disorientation of,
　　100, 118
　mental lapses of, 120, 130
　misinformation about, 144–145
　patient rights, advocating for,
　　146–150
　symptoms of, 12, 13, 16, 18, 28,
　　32, 52, 136
Multiple Sclerosis Education
　Network, 143

Natalizumab, 170
National Multiple Sclerosis Society
　(NMSS), 27, 28, 92, 106, 107,
　109, 112, 146, 147, 195, 198
neurologist, 22, 28, 64, 108, 149,
　183, 196
Neurology Clinic, University
　of Wisconsin-Madison, 33

neuropsychological testing, 45
neuropsychologist, 44
NMSS. *See* National Multiple
    Sclerosis Society
numbness, 37, 75, 97. *See also*
    steroid treatments

occupational therapy (OT),
    97–99
Open Door magazine, 188–192
optic neuritis, 36, 39. *See also*
    vision problems
oral medication, 34

painkillers, 78
Peer Supporter volunteers,
    106–107, 108, 110, 146–150
personal digital assistants (PDAs)
    for memory assistance,
    100–101
Pettit National Ice Center,
    33, 181
physical therapy (PT), 97–99, 117
PML. *See* Progressive multifocal
    leukoencephalopathy
Post-Its™, 102, 139
progressive diseases, 32, 37
progressive multifocal
    leukoencephalopathy (PML),
    170–172, 174

Rebif®, 168, 169, 171, 175
recognition problems, familiar
    people/places, 129–137
referrals to medical
    professionals, 48
resources, 201–204
retirement
    facing, 83–84
    from work, 80–83, 114

safety
    issues, 128
    person, 158–162
seizures and MS, 123
self-education, 196–197
side effects of MS medications, 42,
    73–74, 78–79
social restriction, because of
    symptoms, 54–55
Social Security
    benefits, 81
    Disability, 27
Southgate Mall, 2
speech and language problems,
    140–141
statistics on MS, xv
Staying Smart and Staying Afloat,
    188–192
steroid treatments, 37, 75–76, 97
stress, 10
    and MS exacerbations, 61, 83
subcutaneous injection, 168
sunglasses, 39. *See also* vision
    problems
support groups, 27–28
support systems, family and friends
    as, 59–60, 81–82, 135–137, 197
symptoms of MS, 12, 13, 16, 18,
    28, 32, 52, 64, 136

Tai Chi, 102
taste perception, alterations in, 37
team efforts, 165–179
temper outbursts, 56–58. *See also*
    anger management
therapy program, 99
tips for living, 12, 25, 38–39,
    48–49, 83–84, 96, 113–115,
    128, 142, 150–151, 162–163,
    178–179, 193

TOUCH Prescribing Program, 172, 173
traveling, 187–192
treatment. *See* medications for MS
trilevel program, 183
Tylenol®, 73
Tysabri®, 169–178, 192

United Performing Arts Fund (UPAF), 90, 92
UPAF. *See* United Performing Arts Fund

Vandlik, Renee, 146–147
virus, 16, 17
  JC virus, 171
vision problems, 13–15, 17–19, 31–32, 36, 39. *See also* optic neuritis

vitamin D as treatment for MS, 33–34
volunteering, 81, 103–110, 146–147

web sites for MS support, 110–111, 203–204
wellness, 181–187
  fitness program, 183
wheelchair
  mental, drifting and dragging in, 129–142
"wheelchair stick factor," 1
word-finding problems, 140–141
workouts
  energize, 183
  maximize, 183
  vitalize (chair-based), 183
yoga, 102